Attention-Deficit Hyperactivity Disorder

a natural way to treat ADHD

Attention-Deficit Hyperactivity Disorder

a natural way to treat ADHD

Professor Basant K. Puri

MA (Cantab), PhD, MB, BChir, BSc (Hons)
MathSci, MRCPsych, DipStat, MMath

Consultant/Professor, MRI Unit,
Imaging Sciences Department,
MRC Clinical Sciences Centre, Hammersmith Hospital, London
and Head of the Lipid Neuroscience Group,
Imperial College London

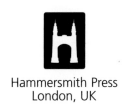

Hammersmith Press
London, UK

First published in 2005 by Hammersmith Press Limited,
496 Fulham Palace Road, London SW6 6JD, UK

© Hammersmith Press Limited 2005

British Library Cataloguing in Publication Data: A CIP record of this book is available
from the British Library.

ISBN 1-905140-01-0
Designed by Julie Delf
Production by Helen Whitehorn, Pathmedia
Illustrations by Jo Knowles
Printed and bound by J.W. Arrowsmith
Cover image: Jacqui Hurst/CORBIS

Contents

1

A Significant Major Breakthrough

Eighteen-year-old Henrietta was referred to me in 2004. The symptoms she described were the classic symptoms of attention-deficit hyperactivity disorder, or 'ADHD'. She complained that she could not concentrate. 'I couldn't play with my toys when I was younger. Now I can't even watch a movie all the way through. I get bored. I fidget and start playing with my 'phone. So I get up and go and get some food.'

When she was still at school, Henrietta had great difficulty coping with her schoolwork. As she described it, 'I could sit in my room for hours and not touch my work. Instead I'd just think of other things to do. I would just argue with my parents and not do my homework.'

At the age of thirteen-and-a-half years, Henrietta, whose family do not live in the United Kingdom, was taken by her parents to see a psychiatrist in England. Let Henrietta take up the account: 'Dr ... [the psychiatrist] made a diagnosis of ADHD. He started me on Ritalin at the age of thirteen-and-a-half. But I developed asthma at fourteen, and I stopped the Ritalin.' I asked her how she had felt while taking the Ritalin (the 'trade' name for a powerful drug, methylphenidate). 'It made me moody. I didn't want to take it. But it did help me to concentrate. I could tell when it was wearing off as well.'

On being probed further about her relationship with her parents, Henrietta readily admitted that she was aware of routinely over-reacting. 'I shout abuse at my parents. Because, say for example mum washes my stuff and then forgets where the things are.' After shouting and swearing at her parents, she would realize she had over-reacted, but only after the event. 'Then I'll think, Henrietta you stupid cow.'

I asked Henrietta for her full medical history and did a physical examination to make sure she had no other serious illness. This process revealed several symptoms and 'signs' that indicated Henrietta might be seriously low in the group of essential nutrients called fatty acids. (For medical doctors, 'symptoms' are the features of a condition that are experienced by the patient, whereas 'signs' are those features that the doctor elicits from the patient. For example, if a patient tells me about feeling tired, then this is a symptom, while if I observe that my patient looks anaemic when I examine them, then that is a sign elicited by me.)

Henrietta suffered from dry skin; indeed, she complained of suffering from 'horrible spots' on her face. Her lips were dry; in fact, she felt she had always had dry lips. Her nails were unusually soft and brittle. She complained that they broke easily, and as if to prove the point, she was able to hold up a broken fingernail. She had an allergy, which resulted in her asthma. She also admitted she regularly had to get up once in the middle of the night to pass water. This phenomenon, known as nocturia in medicine, may be relatively common when one is in one's mid-eighties, but not at eighteen-and-a-half. I would expect to find all these symptoms and signs in someone too low in the fatty acids omega-3 and omega-6 (of which more later in the book). I thought I should therefore explore what might be stopping Henrietta's body from making these fatty acids, as well as what she was actually eating and drinking. She denied taking any illicit drugs or smoking, but she did admit that she would binge drink every Friday and Saturday night with friends. As large amounts of alcohol may get in the way of our cells' ability to manufacture the most important long-chain omega-3 and omega-6 fatty acids from their basic forms in our diet this was important. (Why will be explained in Chapters 4 and 5.)

Caffeine may also prevent our bodies making the important omega-3 and omega-6 fatty acids. While Henrietta did not drink coffee and only drank tea occasionally, she admitted to drinking a massive five to six cans of a diet cola drink every day. I say massive because this represents a large intake of caffeine, of around 250 milligrams (that is, 50 milligrams per can). In comparison, tea contains about 30-50 milligrams of caffeine per cup depending on how it is brewed.

Diet cola is also strongly acidic. Strongly acidic carbonated drinks are not good for our bodies. For example, they often contain phosphoric acid, which prevents our bodies dealing properly with calcium. In turn, this can weaken our bones. However, at least Henrietta did not regularly drink any other fizzy drinks.

For breakfast Henrietta would eat either a bacon sandwich and scrambled eggs or else a sausage sandwich. Then mid-morning she would typically snack on a mixture of crisps, chocolate and sweets. Lunch consisted of either chips, or a turkey and ham sandwich, together with yet more crisps. During the afternoon, Henrietta would again snack each day on crisps, chocolate and sweets. The evening meal depended on whether or not she was eating at home (where she lived with her parents). If dining at home, she would eat the family meal prepared by her health-conscious mother. This would usually consist of either chicken or meat with vegetables or else a pasta dish. Pudding consisted of fruit. (When she told me this, I almost breathed a sigh of relief, as I had been wondering how on earth she was getting important vitamins and minerals. Unfortunately, my relief was short-lived; Henrietta explained that she did not usually eat the fruit.) If she was not eating at home, then her evening meal would consist of her favourite Chinese take-away of beef in black bean sauce with mushrooms and 'special fried rice'.

So here I was, in the twenty-first century, interviewing a young woman from a well-to-do and health-conscious family living in an affluent Western European country who was surviving on an impoverished diet. A significant proportion of her calorie intake each day came from the consumption of three bags of crisps. Crisps are made by deep frying wafer-thin slices of potato at a high temperature in oil. One result of the cooking conditions is that some of the fatty acids in the vegetable oil are turned into artificial 'trans' fats (see Chapter 5). Our bodies did not evolve to be able to cope with large quantities of such fats. Sadly, some of the delicate and intricate biochemical and physiological mechanisms of the human body are fooled into absorbing these trans fats and inserting them into the brain and other organs in place of the missing omega-3 and omega-6 fatty acids. Some of the results of this are explained later in the book.

Henrietta also ate a lot of refined white sugar in the chocolate, sweets and fizzy drinks. Again, our bodies did not develop to cope with large quantities of this seemingly innocent yet actually powerful substance. Too much refined sugar can have profound effects on a person's mood, to say nothing of the adverse consequences for their physical well-being. Incidentally, the chocolates being rich in hydrogenated vegetable oil, were another source of trans fats in her diet. (This is not true of chocolate made by companies such as Green & Black, which are low in trans fats. The ingredient to avoid in chocolate or any other product is 'vegetable fat' or more specifically 'hydrogenated vegetable fat'.) The chocolates were also an additional source of caffeine, dark chocolate not surprisingly being higher in caffeine than milk chocolate. (An American study found that a popular brand of milk chocolate contains 10 milligrams caffeine per 1.5 ounces, while a popular dark chocolate contains 31 milligrams per 1.5 ounces.) The special fried rice and the chips provided yet more manufactured trans fats. The sweets and Chinese black bean sauce were also a rich source of artificial colourings. She ate no oily fish at all and almost no fresh fruit. It was little wonder that she was seriously low in certain important fatty acids and that she complained of always feeling tired.

It was time for me to make my recommendations for treatment. I invited one of Henrietta's parents to join us. First, I confirmed that I agreed with the diagnosis of ADHD. Then I explained that Henrietta was too low in important long-chain omega-3 and omega-6 fatty acids and also probably too low in several important vitamins and minerals that help the body as 'cofactors'. (What this means is explained more fully in Chapter 8.) Furthermore, her consumption of manufactured trans fats, caffeine, artificial colourings and refined sugar was just far too high. (Ideally, these should be close to zero.) I recommended that Henrietta immediately begin to take a supplement that contains a combination of pure EPA (an extremely important long-chain omega-3 fatty acid), virgin evening primrose oil (an excellent source of both omega-6 fatty acids and triterpines), and absolutely zero DHA. (At the time of this book going to press there is only one supplement available, called VegEPA, that provides exactly this combination and which has been tested in both the laboratory and in patients. Later in this book you will see why this combination is so important. The reason is complicated, but I have explained it as clearly as I can and I have provided a Glossary at the end of the book where you can look up terms such as DHA.)

I recommended that Henrietta take eight capsules of this supplement a day. I suggested that she take four each morning and four each evening, preferably with food. I explained that this would deliver exactly the correct daily adult doses of the fatty acids she needed. (I also explained that Henrietta should stick with the supplement I recommended for the reasons I've already given. Apparently cheaper alternatives would be a false economy as they would not provide the right combination of ingredients.)

Henrietta asked me if this preparation was like the Ritalin she had unsuccessfully tried five years before. I explained that it was nothing like methylphenidate, but consisted instead purely of naturally occurring substances that were perfectly safe to take. Indeed, I admitted I was taking eight capsules daily myself. (I do not suffer from ADHD. As you will see in Chapter 9, there are considerable other health benefits to be derived from taking pure EPA and virgin evening primrose oil; this is why I take the supplement.) Henrietta felt very reassured and agreed to start taking the fatty acid supplement at the dose recommended by me. When it came to making radical changes to her diet, however, she was far less accommodating. She felt she could not function without her daily diet cola drinks. The crisps, chocolates and sweets were sacrosanct, as was the special fried rice. She did not like the idea of eating fresh fruit, but she did reluctantly agree to drink one or two glasses of freshly squeezed orange juice each day. (Again, as with the supplement, I encouraged her not to try to save money by buying cheaper 'orange juice drinks' available in supermarkets in cartons. These tend to be made from concentrate, and contain a lot of sugar. It is far better to drink real orange juice that has been made by freshly squeezing the fruit.)

While I normally prefer my patients to get their important vitamins and minerals from a rich and varied diet, in this case I had no choice but to recommend a small daily dose of vitamin B complex and certain minerals. (In this case, cheaper is actually often better! I strongly urged them not to buy expensive mega-vitamin or mega-mineral preparations. One excellent possibility would have been that Henrietta take two VegeCO capsules daily; each of these capsules contains just the right combination of vitamins and minerals (see Chapter 8) at safe levels. Unfortunately, VegeCO was not available when I saw Henrietta, and so instead I suggested that she buy an ordinary multi-vitamin and multi-mineral preparation, such as those sold in the United Kingdom by the supermarket group J Sainsbury. The Sainsbury's products do not exceed the Recommended Daily Allowances for the vitamins and minerals they contain.)

I saw Henrietta and her parents three months later. She was a transformed person. Her face looked much healthier. Indeed, she was very pleased with her much improved appearance. The dryness of her lips, which had affected her for years, had almost cleared up. Her nails were now the best they had ever been; she proudly displayed her fingers to me. Wonderful as these physical changes were, they were dwarfed by the improvements in her ADHD symptoms. She could now concentrate better than she had in many years. She was performing really well in her job. Now, not only could she watch a film all the way to the end, without losing track of the main plot and subplots, but she had found that she had just started to enjoy reading for pleasure. The arguments with her parents and the moodiness were no longer features of her life. Her father was very proud of his daughter.

Excitingly, Henrietta's story is one of a growing number. As a result of a recent major breakthrough in research, there is, at long last, excellent news for people whose lives are devastated by ADHD. This is good news, not just for those who suffer from this debilitating illness and their immediate carers, but also for their wider families, friends, teachers, and schoolmates or work-mates. Starting around the year 2000, an international group of medical researchers and neuroscientists investigating medical disorders, has produced a significant body of research, which at last heralds a major advance in the treatment of ADHD. This group includes in particular two British researchers, Dr Alex Richardson and myself, the author of this book.

By studying the way in which our bodies work at the most basic level, the level of the millions of molecules that make us up, and by carefully observing the responses of patients in my clinical and research practices, we have discovered increasing evidence for an exciting new approach. We have found that the combination of two naturally occurring substances, in the right ratio, as taken by Henrietta, can significantly improve the symptoms of ADHD, even in its most severe form.

The first of these substances is a particular fatty acid found in nature, and known in the medical and scientific community by the rather long-winded name eicosapentaenoic acid (EPA). The second substance is virgin evening primrose oil (virgin EPO). And this combination works best when there is a complete *absence* of another fatty acid called docosahexaenoic acid (DHA). Why this regime should work, the detailed evidence for its usefulness, and how to follow it will all be explained within this book.

Our research is backed up by the use of advanced chemical analysis techniques. These confirm there are low levels of impor-tant fatty acids in people with ADHD. At the time of writing, there have been three medical studies or 'trials' using these natural substances, EPA and EPO – two in the United Kingdom (both involving Dr Richardson and me), and one in the United States of America. All three trials have demonstrated that our particular combination of natural substances is highly effective in treating the symptoms of ADHD.

Up until now, the most common treatment for anyone suffering from this debilitating disease has been powerful stimulating drugs or 'psychostimulants', including drugs that closely resemble amphetamines, even if the patient is only a young child. These psychostimulants can, and do, cause a range of unpleasant side-effects, which are described in Chapter 6. In contrast, the natural treatment option advocated in this book carries with it a range of highly beneficial 'side-effects', which are described in detail in Chapter 9.

Before explaining how this new approach came about I am going to look at the wider picture. How many people have ADHD? What are its causes? How have the psychostimulants come to be the standard treatment up until now? For those of you who simply want practical information on diet and supplements, please do go straight to Chapter 6 and beyond. However, I very much hope you will stay with me to see why the new approach holds out such promise. You may find the going gets tough at times, as I have had to include a fair amount of scientific theory, but all explained step by step.

With any new approach in medicine, scientific credibility is very important. Throughout the book you will find I have included references to articles, especially research papers, which have been published in established scientific journals. All these are listed at the end of the book. Within the text I have used the convention of simply giving the authors' surnames plus the year in which the article was published. Many of these articles can be found on the Web, in summary or in full, if you want to go to the original sources. The reference list at the end of the book will give you all the information you need to find them.

Finally, before I get into the detail of the book, I would like to make a point about the supplements I recommend. I have been criticised for recommending only one fatty acid supplement to the exclusion of all others. I wish I could recommend a range as I think competition is healthy. However, at the present time only one fatty acid supplement has the combination that my research tells me is safe and effective; I would be failing in my duty to my patients not to give them what I believe to be the correct advice.

2

A Wider Perspective

Is ADHD a medical illness?

You may have heard several, possibly contradictory, theories about the causes of ADHD and why more and more people seem to have it. Many have been put forward. I will be considering some of these in detail in Chapter 3.

A number of these theories imply that ADHD is not really a medical illness at all. For instance, some researchers have argued that the main cause of ADHD may be bad parenting. Others put the 'blame' on 'liberal' teaching practices including a lack of appropriate discipline in modern schools. Various social factors have also been put forward as causes. These include the break-up of families and family life, increasingly common now in so many modern societies and made worse by the need for greater geographical mobility in today's job markets. The reduced role of religious belief has also been blamed, together with the loss of the social cohesion that can go hand-in-hand with communal religious practice. More generally, the rise in ADHD has been put down to the way our lives seem to have become more complicated and stressful. Whereas in the 1980s e-mails were a novelty, now it seems as if many of us are enslaved by the need to be able to respond rapidly to an avalanche of communications from e-mails and mobile telephone calls and text messages.

The good news is that the results of our research have shown that this dreadful illness is associated with clear-cut changes in the chemistry of the body. Once these chemical abnormalities are treated, in the completely natural way I shall describe later, the chances are very high that anyone who has ADHD will become better and no longer suffer from this disorder. In other words, our research shows that ADHD really is a medical illness, and one that can be easily treated in a safe way. And if this is the case, it must be unfair to hold hard-pressed parents or teachers responsible for the increasing number of children with this illness.

It is also not right to blame the individual who suffers from ADHD. If a person develops pneumonia, ordinarily we would not consider it appropriate to blame them for their illness. In a similar way, we should adopt a tolerant attitude to children and adults with ADHD, and recognize that their behaviour is the result of a treatable medical problem. Having said that, I have been interested to discover that a psychotherapist, named Georg Groddeck, working in the last century *did* blame pneumonia sufferers for their lung infection! Why, he would ask the patient in therapy, had they allowed themselves to become infected? He even considered that a broken leg might be caused by the patient – perhaps, Groddeck argued, he (or she) had unconsciously allowed himself to fall in order to break a limb. I should point out that many of these and similar ideas of Georg Groddeck, who lived from 1866 to 1934 and was a contemporary of Sigmund Freud, are no longer accepted by modern psychiatrists and psychologists, but the relationship between 'body' and 'mind' in illness remains highly controversial.

ADHD also carries the stigma that is generally associated with mental or psychological illness. The rights and wrongs of this would fill another book. What cannot be denied is how difficult, indeed almost impossible, it can be for some parents to admit that their child is suffering from ADHD because of this stigma. This may be even more of a problem with adults who are ADHD sufferers. In turn, this may make sufferers or their relatives that bit less likely to seek medical help. (In my clinical experience, however, there is often a palpable sense of relief when adults realize that they have been suffering from ADHD for the whole of their lives, extending back to adolescence and childhood.)

Another problem is that people with ADHD and their carers are generally aware that even if they do seek treatment, at the present time this is likely to take the form of drug treatment with powerful psychostimulants such as *Ritalin*, or methylphenidate, the treatment Henrietta had tried and rejected. Many parents of children with ADHD or adult ADHD sufferers simply do not wish to take powerful drugs of this sort, and may not seek help for this reason. Thus it is that, even though there appears to be an inexorable rise in the recorded numbers of new cases of ADHD throughout the world, in reality many people with this condition, and in particular adult sufferers, may not be recognized.

The impact of ADHD

In spite of possible under-diagnosis, ADHD is widely discussed nowadays in newspapers and magazines, and on radio and television. This is hardly surprising given that this illness seems to have been spreading dramatically in many countries, led by the United States of America, over the course of the twentieth century. Many British readers will remember a time when schoolchildren would queue up for their mid-morning free school milk. By the 1990s, there were reports of schools in America in which many children would also have to queue up each school day; this time, they were not queuing for milk, but for their stimulant anti-ADHD medication.

On 16th May 2000, Terrance Woodworth, the Deputy Director of the Office of Diversion Control of the United States Drug Enforcement Administration (or DEA) gave a Congressional Testimony before the 'Committee on Education and the Workforce: Subcommittee on Early Childhood, Youth and Families'. This testimony included some chilling words (reproduced here with official permission from the DEA) about the increased use of psychostimulant medication in the United States during the 1990s.

The DEA is the agency responsible for the regulation and control of substances with abuse potential that are subject to the Controlled Substances Act (CSA). ... In striving to maintain this balance, the DEA has made every effort to keep the health and safety of our young people uppermost in our mind. Of the many psychoactive substances prescribed to young children in the United States, only two controlled substances are widely utilized by American physicians to treat children: methylphenidate (commonly known as Ritalin®) and amphetamine (primarily Adderall® and Dexedrine®). Both are approved and used in the treatment of attention deficit (hyperactivity) disorder referred to as ADHD or ADD. Both of these substances are powerful stimulants that have been in Schedule II of the CSA since 1971. Schedule II of the CSA contains those substances that have the highest abuse potential and dependence profile of all drugs that have medical utility.

In 1995, in response to a petition by Children and Adults With Attention Deficit Disorder (CH.A.D.D.) and the American Academy of Neurology to lower the regulatory controls on methylphenidate, the DEA conducted an extensive review of the use, abuse liability, actual abuse, diversion, and trafficking of methylphenidate. The CH.A.D.D. petition character-ized methylphenidate as a mild stimulant with little abuse potential – this is not what our review found...

The DEA has observed a dramatic increase in the production and use of both methylphenidate and amphetamine. Each year, the DEA establishes an aggregate production quota (APQ) for each Schedule I and II controlled substance. This quota is based on sales and inventory data supplied by the manufacturers as well as information supplied by the Food and Drug Administration (FDA) regarding legitimate medical and research needs. The methylphenidate quota has increased from 1,768 kilograms in 1990 at which time there were two bulk manufac-turers and four dosage-form manufacturers. This year [2000], the APQ is 14, 957 kilograms with six bulk manufacturers and 19 dosage form manufacturers. Prior to 1991, domestic sales reported by the manufacturers of methylphenidate remained stable at approximately 2,000 kilograms per year. By 1999, domestic sales increased by nearly

500 per cent. The amphetamine APQ has increased from 417 kilograms in 1990 with two bulk manufacturers and seven dosage form manufacturers. This year's amphetamine APQ is 9,007 kilograms with six bulk manufacturers and 19 dosage form manufacturers. This is more than a 2,000 per cent increase for amphetamine in nine years (See Figure 1).

The increases in production and use of methylphenidate are even more striking when compared to worldwide data (Figure 2). According to the United Nations, the U.S. produces and consumes about 85 per cent of the world's production of methylphenidate....

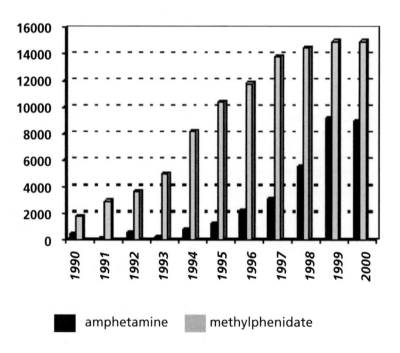

Figure 1. Aggregate Production Quota (kilograms) of amphetamine and methylphenidate. Based on data from the United States Drug Enforcement Agency (DEA). Reproduced with permission from the DEA (www.dea.gov; see www.usdoj.gov/dea/pubs/cngrtest/ct051600.htm)

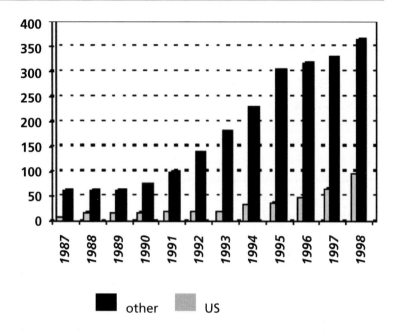

Figure 2. United Nations data relating to methylphenidate consumption. The vertical scale gives the daily dose in millions of prescriptions. Reproduced with permission from the DEA (www.dea.gov; see www.usdoj.gov/dea/pubs/cngrtest/ct051600.htm)

There is an adage that where America leads today, the rest of the Western world follows tomorrow. The huge increase in the prescribed use of psychostimulants in the United States during the 1990s shown in Figures 1 and 2 is reflected by similar increases occurring, after a time lag of a few years, in other Western countries. Overall, the estimates of how widespread ADHD is worldwide vary from 4% of the total population at the low end to an astonishing 19% at the high end (Buitelaar, 2002). Using the more conservative figures, in the United Kingdom NICE (the National Institute for Clinical Excellence) has estimated that ADHD affects around one in twenty, or 5%, of school-age children. Of these 5%, a fifth (that is, 1% of school-age children, about 69,000 six to 16-year-olds in England and 4,200 in Wales) are thought to suffer from a severe form of ADHD called hyperkinetic disorder (National Institute for

Clinical Excellence, 2000). It follows that, in a typical British school class containing 30 pupils, on average one or two children will have ADHD, while on average in every three classes one child will have a severe form of ADHD. Of course, the true figures might be much higher if there are indeed many children who have not been diagnosed as having this condition.

ADHD carries an enormous cost. There are the obvious financial costs of extra specialized staff in schools, of psychological assessments, of psychological interventions, of extra childcare at home, and of children who may end up not fulfilling their true potential in terms of their careers and salaries and all they might contribute to society. The costs are not just financial, though. There are social and emotional costs that can also be heavy. The costs to families and marriages perhaps stressed almost to breaking point (or beyond) by the strain of looking after one or more children with ADHD. The costs to the educational system of having to try to contain disruptive behaviour in the classroom. And then there are the individual medical consequences of the stress on the lives of the parents and teachers who have to look after children with ADHD: premature ageing; reduced resistance to infections and to cancer; and increased risks of heart attacks and strokes, to name but a few.

Drug-company research

The social causes I've mentioned already are not the only reasons put forward for the increasing tide worldwide of ADHD. Modern research, much of which is directly or indirectly sponsored by large pharmaceutical companies, does indicate that this illness has biological causes. In particular, various chemicals in the brain have been found to be abnormal in ADHD, particularly those involved in transmitting information between nerve cells, and therefore known as neurotransmitters. Some of this research is certainly valid. However, as we shall see later in this book, it was the use of psychostimulants that came first. Attempts to provide scientific 'justification' for their use followed after.

Few doubt that the symptoms and signs of ADHD have been helped in many children who have been prescribed these psychostimulants. Unfortunately, these drugs carry the risk of a range of unpleasant side-effects. This is hardly surprising, given that many of the popular ones such as methylphenidate behave in our bodies in much the same way as amphetamines or cocaine. Who would give their child a small dose of an amphetamine or of cocaine and not expect unpleasant reactions?

New synthetic drugs that are non-stimulant are being developed for the treatment of ADHD in children and adolescents. The first to come on the market was Strattera, with the official 'chemical' name atomoxetine hydrochloride. (When a drug is first discovered and manufactured, the company concerned will usually give the drug a 'trade' name, which normally starts with a capital letter. In due course, once the patent for that drug expires, other companies are at liberty to manufacture and sell the drug in its non-patented non-proprietary or 'generic' form. For instance, the drug methylphenidate has been sold for many years under the trade name Ritalin but the patent has now expired and a number of companies supply it under its generic name.) Strattera was approved for use in the treatment of ADHD in children, adolescents and adults in the United States of America by the Food and Drug Administration (FDA) (part of the United States Department of Health and Human Services) on 26th November 2002. However, as explained more fully in Chapter 6, there have been increasing reports of negative side-effects with these new drugs too. In the United Kingdom, the *Daily Telegraph* carried the following article by Celia Hall, their Medical Editor, on 4th February 2005, entitled 'Children's drug can cause liver damage'.

The parents of hyperactive children who take a drug to control their condition were warned yesterday of a possible risk of serious liver damage.

The drug, Straterra [sic] or atomoxetine, was launched in 2002 and became available last summer in Britain for the treatment of attention deficit hyperactivity disorder, ADHD.

In America about two million children and adults have used it while in Britain it has been used by about 10,000 patients to date.

… But yesterday the Medicine and Healthcare Regulatory Agency issued new advice following a review of the drug by [the] Committee o[n] Safety o[f] Medicines (CSM). They said they believed the risk of liver poisoning was one in 50,000.

The American Food and Drug [Administration] issued a similar warning in December. …

Prof Duff added: 'We have advised doctors that if they suspect liver problems are occurring, treatment should be stopped and an alternative treatment initiated.'

… Itchy skin, dark urine, abdominal tenderness, jaundice and unexplained 'flu-like' symptoms can all be a sign of liver problems. In Britain 67 adverse reactions to the drug have been reported by GPs, including three reports of liver problems.

These difficulties with conventional medical drug treatment have made increasing numbers of parents seek alternative remedies. Certainly, 'talking', or more formally 'psychological' treatments can help make some difference, for the good, in many cases. Unfortunately, the waiting lists for good psychologists tend to be very long, while securing the services of a private psychologist over a long period of time can be very expensive. (A psychologist is not to be confused with a psychiatrist. A psychiatrist is a medically qualified doctor who has gone on to specialize in psychiatry and is therefore licensed to prescribe drugs. The vast majority of psychologists, on the other hand, are not medical doctors but have a different qualification licensing them to give a variety of 'talking' treatments.) There is the added problem that, in some countries, psychologists may actually recommend that children be referred to a psychiatrist for treatment with a psychostimulant – the very thing that parents might be trying to avoid in the first place. Some parents have turned to the complementary and alternative medicine sector. Children with ADHD can certainly benefit from changes in their diet that involve avoiding artificial colourings, such as tartrazine, and sweeteners. Other changes in diet that can help will be described in chapters 8 and 10 of this book. However, until our research was carried out, there was never any scientifically convincing evidence that any of the alternative treatments actually worked.

3

What is ADHD?

After coming across attention-deficit hyperactivity disorder as a medical student, my formal introduction to this illness in children and adolescents came when I was working as a junior doctor in child and adolescent psychiatry. I was fortunate to be working under an outstanding clinician named Dr Paul Laking, who was a simply brilliant teacher. (Together with another exceptionally gifted clinician, Dr Ian Treasaden, we would go on to write our successful *Textbook of Psychiatry*, which came out in its second edition in 2003. The excellent chapter entitled Child and Adolescent Psychiatry in this book was, naturally enough, written by Paul Laking and is warmly recommended to the interested reader. Sadly, Paul died in January 2005.)

Under the guidance of Dr Laking, I learned how to recognize the three cardinal features of ADHD and see at first hand how this illness can co-exist with other disorders. I am going to describe these and other related aspects of ADHD in this chapter.

Cardinal features

Anyone who lives or works with children, adolescents or adults suffering from ADHD is struck by the way the three fundamental features of the illness appear. These features are 'inattention', 'hyperactivity' and 'impulsivity'. Not all cases of ADHD are the same. Different levels of each of these three features can appear in different individual sufferers, and, within each feature, there will likely be differences in the type and/or degree of the symptoms and signs.

Inattention

The hallmark of 'inattention' is brief and changing activities. (In fact, it could be argued that the term inattention is not necessarily the best name for this.) For instance, a child or adult with ADHD may have difficulty in following a set of tasks properly and completing an activity. A schoolchild may find it difficult to complete his or her homework, like Henrietta (see Chapter 1). Adults may have difficulty finishing their duties at work. In fact, they may be reluctant to get involved in any task that requires sustained mental effort. Even reading a book may be too hard.

People with ADHD often make careless mistakes. They may not pay enough attention to details. When spoken to they may appear not to be listening properly. Trying to organize an activity that involves them can prove to be a nightmare for them and their carers, families or work colleagues. They may also be distracted very easily, and generally be rather forgetful.

Hyperactivity

Hyperactivity, or over activity, is another key feature of ADHD. People with the condition often fidget around and may not be able to sit still. They may run around when this is not appropriate. Parents can become very worried seeing their children with ADHD running along pavements apparently blissfully unaware of other pedestrians and the risk from road traffic. Schoolteachers can find it disruptive to have children in their class who keep leaving their seats inappropriately.

Some adolescents and adults with ADHD talk about how they feel driven and how they are always 'on the go'. This may be mirrored by speech that seems incessant and sometimes difficult to interrupt.

Clearly, whether or not any particular behaviour is an example of over activity or hyperactivity depends on its context. While running at speed on a pavement or across a road is not normal, unless you are about to miss your bus, the same action on a football pitch may be highly commendable (though not, of course, if you are running the wrong way).

Impulsivity

The third fundamental or 'core' feature of ADHD, 'impulsivity' may show itself as difficulty in waiting in turn in a queue, say, or interrupting others inappropriately.

One of my colleagues, Jonathan, realized he had ADHD after hearing my description of the condition at one of my lectures. He excitedly rushed up to me after the lecture and told me that his whole life now made sense as he could see that he had all the hallmark symptoms and signs of ADHD. (The criteria for this diagnosis are included later in this chapter.) For example, he could now understand why it was that he could never give a lecture without becoming easily distracted by irrelevant things. Also, while attending lectures, he had a habit of blurting out his thoughts while the lecturer might be in the middle of developing his argument. He also understood now why he had problems at work. Jonathan was kind enough to give me a lift in his car that day. Unfortunately, after dropping me off at the railway station, partly as a result of his ADHD, including inattention and impulsivity, he promptly went on to have a car crash, though luckily he was not hurt. Jonathan agreed to start taking a fatty acid supplement containing pure EPA, virgin evening primrose oil and no DHA. Within six weeks we all noticed how much calmer and more focused he had become. Even his employers remarked on his excellent progress.

Diagnostic criteria

In general, the criteria used by doctors and psychologists when making a diagnosis of ADHD 'clinically' (for the purposes of patient care alone) are not as strict as the criteria used when carrying out a research project. There are several reasons for this. One is that for a research study it is important to make the group of patients being studied as uniform as possible in terms of their symptoms and signs. This helps researchers to compare like with like when examining the results of different studies.

There are two major sets of diagnostic criteria in common use in the ADHD research community, one published by the American Psychiatric Association, and the other by the World Health Organization. I am going to describe these now.

American Psychiatric Association

The American Psychiatric Association has developed strict diagnostic criteria, which are the first choice of many researchers, including me. The latest diagnostic offering (at the time of writing) is to be found within the Association's *Diagnostic and Statistical Manual of Mental Disorders, fourth edition, Text Revision*. This was published in 2000, and is usually abbreviated to DSM-IV-TR.

The DSM-IV-TR criteria for ADHD (actually, for 'attention-deficit/hyperactivity disorder') are shown in Box 1. As you can see they include a lot of different options, reflecting how much the symptoms of ADHD can vary between one individual and another.

Box 1. DSM-IV-TR diagnostic criteria for attention-deficit/ hyperactivity disorder (Reprinted with permission from The Diagnostic and Statistical Manual of Mental Disorders, copyright 2000. American Psychiatric Association.)

A. Either (1) or (2):
  (1) six (or more) of the following symptoms of **inattention** have persisted for at least 6 months to a degree that is maladaptive and inconsistent with developmental level:
  Inattention
    (a) often fails to give close attention to details or makes careless mistakes in schoolwork, work, or other activities
    (b) often has difficulty sustaining attention in tasks or play activities
    (c) often does not seem to listen when spoken to directly
    (d) often does not follow through on instructions and fails to finish schoolwork, chores, or duties in the workplace (not due to oppositional behavior or failure to under-stand instructions)

(e) often has difficulty organizing tasks and activities
(f) often avoids, dislikes, or is reluctant to engage in tasks that require sustained mental effort (such as school work or homework)
(g) often loses things necessary for tasks or activities (e.g., toys, school assignments, pencils, books, or tools)
(h) is often easily distracted by extraneous stimuli
(i) is often forgetful in daily activities

(2)   six (or more) of the following symptoms of **hyperactivity-impulsivity** have persisted for at least 6 months to a degree that is maladaptive and inconsistent with developmental level:

Hyperactivity
(a) often fidgets with hands or feet or squirms in seat
(b) often leaves seat in classroom or in other situations in which remaining seated is expected
(c) often runs about or climbs excessively in situations in which it is inappropriate (in adolescents or adults, may be limited to subjective feelings of restlessness)
(d) often has difficulty playing or engaging in leisure activities quietly
(e) is often "on the go" or often acts as if "driven by a motor"
(f) often talks excessively

Impulsivity
(g) often blurts out answers before questions have been completed
(h) often has difficulty awaiting turn
(i) often interrupts or intrudes on others (e.g., butts into conversations or games)

B. Some hyperactive-impulsive or inattentive symptoms that caused impairment were present before age 7 years.

C. Some impairment from the symptoms is present in two or more settings (e.g., at school [or work] and at home).

D. There must be clear evidence of clinically significant impairment in social, academic, or occupational functioning.

E. The symptoms do not occur exclusively during the course of a Pervasive Developmental Disorder, Schizophrenia, or other Psychotic Disorder and are not better accounted for by another mental disorder...

World Health Organization

The World Health Organization has its own diagnostic criteria for mental and behavioural disorders. The tenth revision of its *International Classification of Diseases* was published in 1992 and is known as ICD-10. The ICD-10 criteria are not as strict as those of DSM-IV-TR, which is one reason why they are often not used in ADHD research.

The ICD-10 criteria for ADHD (actually, for 'hyperkinetic disorders') are listed in Box 2. These are really diagnostic guidelines, rather than the stricter 'operationally-defined' criteria of DSM-IV-TR shown in Box 1.

Box 2. ICD-10 Diagnostic guidelines for hyperkinetic disorders (Reproduced from the ICD-10 Classification of Mental and Behavioural Disorders: Clinical Descriptions and Diagnostic Guidelines, Geneva, WHO1992, with permission).

The cardinal features are impaired attention and overactivity: both are necessary for the diagnosis and should be evident in more than one situation (e.g. home, classroom, clinic).

Impaired attention is manifested by prematurely breaking off from tasks and leaving activities unfinished. The children change frequently from one activity to another, seemingly losing interest in one task because they become diverted to another... These deficits in persistence and attention should be diagnosed only if they are excessive for the child's age and IQ.

Overactivity implies excessive restlessness, especially in situations requiring relative calm. It may, depending upon the situation, involve the child running and jumping around, getting up from a seat when he or she was supposed to remain seated, excessive talkativeness and noisiness, or fidgeting and wriggling. The standard for judgement should be that the activity is excessive in the context of what is expected in the situation and by comparison with other children of the same age and IQ. This behavioural feature is most evident in structured, situations that require a high degree of behavioural self-control.

The associated features are not sufficient for the diagnosis or even necessary, but help to sustain it. Disinhibition in social

---

relationships, recklessness in situations involving some danger, and impulsive flouting of social rules (as shown by intruding on or interrupting others' activities, prematurely answering questions before they have been completed, or difficulty in waiting turns) are all characteristic of children with this disorder.

… The characteristic behaviour problems should be of early onset (before age 6 years) and long duration. However, before the age of school entry, hyperactivity is difficult to recognize because of the wide normal variation: only extreme levels should lead to a diagnosis in preschool children.

Diagnosis of hyperkinetic disorder can still be made in adult life. The grounds are the same, but attention and activity must be judged with reference to developmentally appropriate norms…

Gender differences

In Chapter 2 we looked briefly at the figures relating to how common ADHD is. There is another aspect to this, and that is the apparent difference in how common ADHD is between males and females. In outpatient clinics, the ratio of boys with ADHD to girls is typically around nine to one. This does not necessarily mean that nine times as many boys suffer from ADHD as girls. Many doctors believe that girls with ADHD are less likely to be referred to specialist clinics than boys. Some teachers reckon that girls tend to be identified at a later age than boys, which would also skew the apparent ratio in favour of boys. A recent American survey by Dr Patricia Quinn and Dr Sharon Wigal, published in 2004, also found that almost half of teachers felt that girls were less likely to 'act out' while a fifth agreed that girls are generally more obedient than boys.

Commenting on the different way girls with ADHD show signs of their condition, Quinn and Wigal (2004) wrote:

There is also evidence that ADHD takes a different type of toll on girls versus on boys. Although they do not differ from boys in measures of impulsivity, school performance, or social interactions, they have greater cognitive and attentional impairment and may be rejected more often by their peers (particularly if they have the inattentive subtype). Needing to repeat a grade in school is also more common among girls than among boys, which supports the observation that they experience more cognitive and academic problems. In a study of adults, females with ADHD showed a higher prevalence of depression, anxiety, and conduct disorder when compared with a control population, as well as cognitive impairments and academic problems. The heavy social and personal impact of ADHD on females points to the importance of early identification and treatment.

...The findings of this survey suggest that gender has important implications for the diagnosis and treatment of ADHD.Among the most striking results is the belief that ADHD often goes unrecognized in girls, a viewpoint broadly held by the general public as well as those who are most familiar with the daily realities of the condition: the parents and teachers of affected children. It was also widely perceived that ADHD presents differently in girls from in boys, and that this is a likely reason for missed or delayed diagnoses in girls. Symptoms such as inattentiveness, poor school performance, and depressive affect are seen as the hallmark signs of ADHD in girls, yet they elicit less attention from teachers and parents than characteristic ADHD symptoms seen in boys, such as disruptive behavior and 'acting out.' This is partly because girls' symptoms are not recognized as typical indications of ADHD and partly because these symptoms are less noticeable and less troublesome to adults than are boys' symptoms. The tendency of girls to 'suffer silently' often means that they bear the burden of untreated ADHD for a much longer time than do boys.

Almost half of the teachers surveyed say that it is harder for them to recognize ADHD symptoms in girls than in boys, and most say they do not have adequate training about the disorder in general. They report that most schools provide little or no training on ADHD for teachers – in fact, only 10% of schools are reported to provide significant training for teachers to learn about ADHD. Even when teachers suspect a child may have ADHD, only half say they inform a child's parent or guardian. For girls with ADHD, this may be because the teachers are unsure of their opinion or because they are concerned that the girls will feel embarrassed or stigmatized by the diagnosis. Reprinted with permission from Medscape General Medicine 6(2), 2004 http://www.medscape.com/viewarticle/472415 (c) 2004 Medscape.

In spite of these differences, there is still evidence that ADHD is more common in boys. The most up-to-date figures for the male to female ratio in the community suggest that boys are about two-and-a-half times as likely as girls to suffer from ADHD. I will describe one reason why this might be the case in Chapter 5 (see page 90).

Development over time

As they get older, children with ADHD come across different kinds of problems as a result of their disorder.

At the age of three or four years, they do not usually have much understanding of how dangerous some activities are. As a result, they are at risk of being hurt accidentally while being inattentive, hyperactive or impulsive. This can be a time of great stress for their parents, as they worry about possible accidents, or have to ferry their children to and from casualty with yet more injuries. Keeping a close eye on your ADHD child can be physically and mentally exhausting.

On starting school, children encounter a new set of challenging environments, including the classroom, school dining hall, assembly hall and playground. The schoolchild with ADHD may find it difficult to sit still in class and not interrupt the teacher. Even the playground can prove to be a problem; a child with ADHD may not be able to play games that involve co-operation. It can be difficult for such a child to make friends or maintain friendships. Academically, children with ADHD are less likely to reach their full potential. Indeed, their school reports are likely to include phrases such as 'Could do better', 'Needs to try harder', 'Must listen more carefully', and 'Must concentrate more in lessons'.

Entry into secondary school (at the age of 11 years in the United Kingdom) is associated with further challenges. The way in which pupils learn gradually shifts in secondary school to more independent study. It is difficult for many schoolchildren with ADHD to deal with this, as in the case of Henrietta (in the first chapter) who could not concentrate on her homework. Many children with ADHD fall even further behind academically.

It is helpful for parents to remember that children of school age only spend around 17% of their time in school. While school is very important, what goes on at home and as part of interactions with other family members will have at least as important an effect on the development of children with ADHD; this needs to be taken into consideration when trying to improve a child's academic performance.

Differentiating ADHD from other disorders

When diagnosing ADHD, it is important that the physician, psychiatrist or psychologist considers the possibility that their patient might be suffering from a different disorder.

One possibility to consider is autism or 'autism spectrum disorder'. (The term 'spectrum disorder' refers to the fact that the features of autism can present in a wide range, or spectrum, of combinations and severities; related to this is the fact that autism is one of a spectrum of closely associated disorders, including ADHD, dyslexia and dyspraxia, as explained below.) For this reason, the specialist must look for the types of problem that occur in autism spectrum disorder. Simply being hyperactive does not necessarily rule out the possibility that the patient suffers from autism spectrum disorder.

Alternatively, hyperactivity and inattention in children may be caused by an anxiety disorder or by depression. Restlessness and agitation can occur as a result of anxiety or depression so a diagnosis of ADHD cannot be based on these two features without first ruling out an emotional disorder.

Hyperactivity can also be the first sign of certain brain disorders, such as adrenoleucodystrophy. (This is a genetic disease that almost exclusively affects males in which there are abnormalities of the outer layer (cortex) of the adrenal glands and the white matter of the brain.) A good medically trained specialist should be able to exclude these.

Perhaps one of the most difficult alternative diagnoses that needs to be excluded is a conduct disorder. Conduct disorders consist of repeated and persistent patterns of antisocial, aggressive or defiant behaviour which exceed what you would normally expect in a child of the same age. Neither toddler tantrums nor isolated episodes of antisocial behaviour are included as conduct disorders. In younger children, particularly at a preschool age, it can sometimes be difficult to tell whether failing to carry out activities is caused by the inattention of ADHD or by the defiance of a conduct disorder. The genetic influences in conduct disorder and ADHD overlap, and conduct disorder ('oppositional defiant' and 'conduct disorders') commonly occur in hyperactivity. Many leading researchers suggest that perhaps the diagnoses of ADHD and conduct disorder should not be seen as being mutually exclusive, or even as 'comorbid' conditions (see below), but rather that conduct disorder may be a complication of ADHD.

Co-existence of other disorders

We have just seen that emotional disorders, that is, anxiety and depression, and conduct disorders, may need to be properly differentiated from ADHD by a specialist. There is a further twist to diagnosing ADHD, which can make the task even more difficult: anxiety, depression or a conduct disorder often actually co-exist with ADHD. This phenomenon is known by doctors as 'comorbidity'.

Another set of disorders that tend to co-exist with ADHD are specific learning difficulties or language difficulties, including dyslexia. These can make it even more difficult for children with ADHD to cope at school. Indeed, reading skills are often delayed in children with ADHD.

Commonly, problems with movement, or 'motor', co-ordination also co-exist with ADHD. Known officially in DSM-IV-TR as 'developmental coordination disorder', another term is 'dyspraxia', which in turn used to be known as 'minimal brain damage' and 'clumsy child syndrome'. In this condition the organization of movement is impaired or develops more slowly than normal. As a result a child may be unable to throw and catch a ball properly at an age when other non-dyspraxic children can do so with ease. This example illustrates yet another reason why children with ADHD, suffering also from dyspraxia, often find it difficult to make friends in the playground.

Children with dyspraxia often have poor handwriting, which can hold back their academic achievement even further. They may also have difficulties with reading and spelling, which will again clearly contribute to poor achievement in class. As a further blow to their confidence, they may have trouble with bedwetting as a result of delayed bladder control.

One of the world's leading experts on dyspraxia is my colleague Dr Madeleine Portwood, of Durham, England. She has produced an excellent manual that can be used by parents concerned that their child might have dyspraxia. This is *Developmental Dyspraxia: Identification and Intervention: A Manual for Parents and Professionals*. (Full details can be found in the References at the end of this book.) Dr Portwood's summary of the main early indications of dyspraxia is as follows:

- Irritable and difficult to comfort – from birth

- Feeding difficulties: milk allergies, colic, restricted diet

- Sleeping difficulties: problems establishing routine, requires constant adult reassurance

- Delayed early motor development: sitting unaided, rolling from side to side; do not usually go through the crawling stage

- High levels of motor activity: constantly moving arms and legs

- Repetitive behaviours: head-banging or rolling

- Sensitive to high levels of noise

- Continued problems with development of feeding skills

- Toilet training may be delayed

- Avoids constructional toys such as jigsaws and Lego®

- Delayed language development: single words not evident until aged three years

- Highly emotional: easily distressed, frequent outbursts of uncontrolled behaviour

- Concentration limited to two or three minutes on any task.

Dr Madeleine Portwood's summary of the signs of dyspraxia in preschool children between the ages of three and five years is as follows:

- Very high levels of motor activity

- Very excitable

- Moves awkwardly

- Difficulty pedalling tricycle or similar toy

- Continues to be messy eater

- Avoids constructional toys such as jigsaws and Lego®

- Poor fine motor skills

- Lack of imaginative play

- Isolated in peer group

- Laterality (left- or right-handed) still not established

- Language difficulties persist

- Sensitive to sensory stimulation (sound, sight, touch)

- Limited response to verbal instructions, and

- Limited concentration.

What do these signs mean in real life? Very high levels of movement, or 'motor activity' can show up in many ways, such as excessive foot-swinging and foot-tapping while seated and engaged in other activities (such as reading or writing), excessive and inappropriate hand-clapping or hand-twisting, or an inability to stay in one place for more than five minutes at a time. Being very excitable may mean the child has temper tantrums, or speaks with a loud and shrill voice. Being easily distressed may also be a form of over-excitability. Moving awkwardly may mean the child is constantly bumping into objects and/or falling. It may also mean making 'mirror movements', with hands flapping when running or jumping. The accident-prone child may frequently fall off his tricycle.

Preschool children who 'continue to be messy eaters' often spill liquid from drinking cups and may prefer to use their fingers to feed themselves. Signs of poor movement control, or 'motor skills' in this age group include difficulty with gripping a pencil or pen properly, difficulty in using a pair of scissors correctly, and drawings that are immature for the child's age. As already mentioned, handwriting might be poor for their age. Children with dyspraxia rarely go in for creative play and typically do not enjoy dressing up or playing appropriately in the home corner or in a Wendy House. Those preschool children who are isolated in their peer group tend to prefer the company of adults. The persistence of language difficulties may mean that the child is referred to a speech therapist. 'Sensitivity to sensory stimulation' can show up as sensitivity to high levels of noise, disliking being touched, or even disliking wearing new clothes. A limited response to verbal instructions can mean that the preschool child with dyspraxia takes longer to respond and may have problems comprehending what they are being asked to do. As a result of limited concentration, the child may often leave tasks uncompleted.

The American Psychiatric Association's DSM-IV-TR *(Diagnostic and Statistical Manual of Mental Disorders, fourth edition, Text Revision)* criteria for 'developmental coordination disorder' are shown in Box 3. These will be referred to again later in this chapter and also in Chapter 5 when I discuss a major clinical study in children with developmental coordination disorder and ADHD involving Dr Madeleine Portwood, Shelagh Lowerson and me.

Box 3. DSM-IV-TR diagnostic criteria for developmental coordination disorder. (Reprinted with permission from the Diagnostic and Statistical Manual of Mental Disorders. Copyright 2000. American Psychiatric Association.)

A.   Performance in daily activities that require motor coordination is substantially below that expected given the person's chronological age and measured intelligence. This may be manifested by marked delays in achieving motor milestones (for example, walking, crawling, sitting), dropping things, "clumsiness," poor performance in sports, or poor handwriting.

B. The disturbance in criterion A significantly interferes with academic achievement or activities of daily living.

C. The disturbance is not due to a general medical condition (for example, cerebral palsy, hemiplegia, or muscular dystrophy) and does not meet criteria for a pervasive developmental disorder.

D. If mental retardation is present, the motor difficulties are in excess of those usually associated with it.

'Tic disorders' may also coexist with ADHD. Tics can take the form of repetitive movements or repetitive sounds. The movements tend to be rapid, are often not under voluntary control, and usually do not follow a specific rhythm. They may take many different forms, such as eye blinking, shoulder shrugging, head shaking, or pulling faces. Vocal tics usually start suddenly and do not serve a specific purpose; they may consist of various swear words and other obscenities being shouted out suddenly. It can be extremely embarrassing for a mother to be walking down a supermarket aisle when, all of a sudden, her ADHD child who also suffers from tics starts to shout out swear words, seemingly at passers-by. Sometimes vocal tics are of a simpler form than words – for example, grunts, squeaks, barks, sniffs, or coughs.

Sadly, some people with ADHD also appear to have a predilection for abusing illegal drugs. These include, in particular, opiates such as heroin, and cocaine. Rates of cigarette smoking and alcohol abuse have also been found to be higher in adolescents and young adults who were diagnosed as ADHD sufferers in childhood. While a straightforward genuine comorbidity may exist between ADHD and substance abuse, the possibility cannot be ruled out that the use of stimulant medications in childhood (such as methylphenidate) may predispose the growing child to using their illegal counterparts when older. Some of these stimulants act in the same way as amphetamine or cocaine and children with ADHD may find they function 'best' when taking these or an illegal counterpart drug such as cocaine, heroin, or crack cocaine. There have certainly been cases of famous singers and film stars who have received psychostimulant medication (sometimes, though not necessarily, for an apparent diagnosis of ADHD) and who have gone on to describe how they can only function when taking cocaine, say. There was a time during the twentieth century when some of the psychiatrists treating glamorous Hollywood stars appeared to have a low threshold for prescribing amphetamines or the psychostimulants used to treat children with ADHD. Some of these famous personalities have sadly gone on to die from overdoses.

Overall, delays in achieving reading skills or proper motor co-ordination can make it increasingly difficult for affected children to socialize. If a seven- or eight-year-old child cannot catch or kick a ball properly or is still wetting their bed, then clearly their self-esteem will also suffer. Besides the problems that the child has, their parents or carers can be overcome by a feeling of utter physical and mental exhaustion. In turn, the child may blame himself or herself if and when their exhausted parents argue.

The name of the disorder

There have been many changes in the official name of the condition which is now referred to as attention-deficit hyperactivity disorder or ADHD. These changes have reflected the varying and shifting emphases given to various components of the disorder.

Minimal brain damage

Minimal brain damage was a name used during the first half of the twentieth century, following the first systematic description, in 1902, of the condition that we would now recognize as ADHD. (This description was written by Professor Sir Frederick Still, and is described in the next chapter.) It was believed at the time to be caused by brain damage (albeit minimal), for example following infection by the organism thought to cause encephalitis lethargica. I shall have more to say about encephalitis lethargica in the next chapter, when discussing the possible cause of ADHD.

Minimal brain dysfunction

By the 1950s the name minimal brain damage had come to be replaced by the term minimal brain dysfunction. The main reason for this change was that no one had been able to to find any evidence of actual brain damage despite using the best techniques then available. This term was used in most child psychiatry and developmental paediatrics clinics. It held sway in many parts of the world until the 1980s, although in North America the diagnostic terms published by the American Psychiatric Association gradually took over, particularly in research studies.

From 'hyperactivity of children' to ADHD

The *Diagnostic and Statistical Manual of Mental Disorders* or DSM of the American Psychiatric Association (see earlier in this chapter) has actually used a different name to refer to the condition we now call attention-deficit hyperactivity disorder, with differing diagnostic criteria, in each of its editions. In its first edition, published in 1952, the DSM (DSM-I) referred to this disorder as 'hyperactivity of children'.

The second edition of DSM, DSM-II, published in 1968, referred to the condition as 'hyperkinetic reaction of childhood'. There was an emphasis on overactivity as the cardinal feature.

The third edition of DSM, DSM-III, was published in 1980.

Here, the name was changed again, this time to 'attention deficit disorder'. This reflected North American opinion at the time that the cardinal features were inattention and impulsiveness. The name attention deficit disorder is the source of the (now historical) abbreviation ADD that you may see if you read some of the older scientific and medical literature about attention-deficit hyperactivity disorder. Moreover, the definition of attention deficit disorder used in DSM-III was based on the assumption that the inattention might occur independently of hyperactivity. Accordingly, DSM-III offered two major subtypes of attention deficit disorder, namely 'ADD with hyperactivity' and 'ADD without hyperactivity'. These gave rise to the abbreviations ADD/H and ADD/WO, respectively.

The revised version of the third edition of DSM, known as DSM-III-R, was published in 1987. Here, the American Psychiatric Association changed the name again, this time to 'attention deficit hyperactivity disorder', from which came the abbreviation ADHD. Operational criteria were offered using which the practising psychiatrist or psychologist could determine whether or not a patient fulfilled the diagnostic criteria for DSM-III-R attention deficit hyperactivity disorder by going through the published checklist. As mentioned earlier, these operational criteria were particularly helpful for researchers, as they allowed them to harmonize their use of the diagnostic term rather better, so that they were more likely to be comparing like with like.

As already mentioned, the current fourth edition of DSM (DSM-IV, published in 1994, and the text revision DSM-IV-TR published in 2000), use the name 'attention-deficit/hyperactivity disorder', whence the currently used up-to-date abbreviation ADHD. Note that some books and articles still refer to ADD or even to ADD/ADHD. Some refer to it as AD/HD to reflect the solidus ('/') symbol that the American Psychiatric Association have chosen to insert in the name of the disorder in DSM-IV and DSM-IV-TR.

The changing DSM diagnostic criteria make it difficult directly to compare studies of attention-deficit hyperactivity disorder that have been carried out using different DSM diagnoses.

DAMP

The formal definition of attention-deficit hyperactivity disorder (actually 'attention deficit hyperactivity disorder', without the hyphen) in DSM-III-R was preceded by an attempt during the 1970s in Scandinavia to produce formal criteria for the syndrome of 'minimal brain dysfunction'. A large study of minimal brain dysfunction was started by the child neurologist Professor Bengt Hagberg in 1974; Professor Hagberg suggested the possible nature of these criteria in a Swedish paper published in 1975. The concept that emerged recognized the co-existence of attention disorder with problems with motor control (as in developmental coordination disorder, or dyspraxia) and in perception. It was introduced by the famous Swedish Professor Christopher Gillberg. The syndrome came to be known by the acronym DAMP, derived from Deficits in:

- Attention

- Motor control, and

- Perception.

The diagnostic criteria for DAMP are given in Box 4.

Box 4. Diagnostic criteria for DAMP. (Reproduced from Hagberg B (1975) *Minimal brain dysfunction*. Läkartidnivigen, with permission from the publisher and author.)

A. Attention-deficit hyperactivity disorder as defined in DSM-IV (or DSM-IV-TR).

B. Developmental coordination disorder as defined in DSM-IV (or DSM-IV-TR).

C. The condition is not better accounted for by cerebral palsy.

D. The condition is not associated with severe learning disability – that is, the IQ should be higher than about 50.

E. Other diagnostic categories often apply (for example, autism spectrum disorder and depression), but are not required for a diagnosis of DAMP.

The concept of DAMP has been used a lot in Scandinavian research into ADHD. For example, in 1982 Professor Christopher Gillberg and his colleagues published a 'total population study' of almost five thousand six-year-old children attending the public preschools in the city of Göteborg (Gothenburg), looking at the occurrence of deficits in attention, motor skills and perception in those who had minimal brain dysfunction. The concept is still in use in some Scandinavian research.

Left neglect

In 2005, a group of researchers working at the Medical Research Council's Cognition and Brain Sciences Unit in Cambridge, England, published evidence that children who 'miss' objects in their left field of vision may have ADHD (Dobler and colleagues, 2005). This condition is known as 'left neglect', and it can occur in adults following a stroke that affects the right half, or hemisphere, of the brain; objects on the left side are simply ignored, or 'neglected'.

The research, published in the *Journal of Child Psychology and Psychiatry*, involved investigating children of normal intelligence who did not have any brain damage. There were two groups of children who were studied. The first group were normal children, without a diagnosis of ADHD. The second group consisted of children who had been referred to clinical services for their attention problems. The researchers found that, regardless of the children's clinical diagnosis, reduced attention was associated with left neglect.

This finding means that ADHD children (and other children with reduced attention spans) are more likely to miss the beginning of words in languages, such as English, which are read from left to right. This means that they may be more likely to be diagnosed as suffering from dyslexia. The link between dyslexia and ADHD has already been alluded to, and another aspect of this link will be described in the next chapter.

Left neglect might also make affected children more likely to knock things over that are on their left side (and that are therefore being ignored). This might make them appear to be clumsy or to have dyspraxia, as discussed already. Such children may also have a tendency only to write or draw pictures on the right-hand side of pages, and this may be reflected in poorer marks in schoolwork.

It is not known why left neglect has this association with ADHD. One possibility is as follows. The right hemisphere of the human brain is involved in noticing and processing information from objects in our left field of vision. It also has an important role in keeping a person awake and alert. This is particularly so in the case of people who are starting to feel bored. So, the problem with the right cerebral (brain) hemisphere is related to a fundamental problem with attention. In the next, final, section of this chapter, we shall look at this issue of attention in a little more detail

Attention and 'executive functions'

The concept of attention appears to be intuitively easy to understand, at least until it is studied in depth. In order to attend to something – perceptions from the outside world or from inside our bodies or minds – we need to be awake and usually in a relatively alert state. I say 'usually' because it is certainly possible to attend to perceptions without being fully conscious of so doing. For example, a driver might be paying attention to the car radio or to a conversation with a passenger and yet at some level also be attending to what is going on on the road and be able to slow down or brake suddenly if necessary. Again, there is the famous 'cocktail party effect', in which while talking to someone at a party your attention is suddenly tuned in to the mention of your name by some-one some distance away to whose conversational patter you had not previously been paying (conscious) attention.

In order to carry out goal-oriented or purposeful actions, our brains have to engage in higher-level thought processes, or 'cognitive processing', known as 'executive functions'. These executive functions allow us to take into account changing circumstances, by appropriately attending to the world around us and processing the information received in the light of factors such as past experience. We have to be able to move chunks of information – or 'thoughts' if you like – around until we home in on the best way forward that will allow us to achieve our desired goal.

In moving chunks of information (or thoughts) around, our brains need to make use of memory aids. In ADHD, some of these memory processes appear not to work correctly. This is now explained in a little more detail.

One important element in this process of moving information around is what we call 'working memory'. It is a bit like a pad and pencil that in everyday life we might resort to to hold information temporarily while we pay attention to something else. For instance, relatives of patients sometimes come to my public lectures. Their overall goal is to discover the latest safe, nutrition-based treatment options. During the course of a lecture I might be asked about the best supplements available for a given illness. If I give out the relevant name(s) and telephone number(s), the members of the audience will not immediately get out their mobile 'phones and call the number(s). Instead, they will write down the number(s) as a temporary measure. Later that day, or the next morning (if it is an evening lecture) they will retrieve the number(s) and then make the telephone call(s) and order the supplement(s). This process of using the information stored on the piece of paper for quick reference, instead of constantly attending to the numbers, is equivalent to 'working memory'. The piece of paper is just a temporary storage device which can be discarded once it has served its purpose. The information can be transferred, in turn, from the piece of paper to a more permanent memory store, such as a telephone number book or diary. In this case, the more permanent store is analogous to the long-term memory of the brain.

'Working memory' can be broken down further into different elements. The brain has circuitry for its own 'visuospatial scratch-pad' (like a pencil and sketchpad or a to-do list or diary) and its own 'articulatory or phonological loop' (a bit like a memo dictaphone). Together with a 'central executive', which controls attention, this setup is known as the 'working memory model', as shown in Figure 3, and was formulated by Baddeley and Hitch (1974). Working memory is an important aspect of executive function, and involves being able to attend to events for long enough for them to be stored adequately (albeit temporarily) in either the visuospatial scratch-pad or the phonological loop.

In children with ADHD there is, by definition, a lack of adequate attention. In fact, these children appear to be living within a five-second time-frame. This is often too short an interval to allow information to be temporarily stored in the visuospatial scratch-pad or the phonological loop. As a result, working memory is impaired. There is also evidence that executive functions may be impaired too; this may be at least partly because working memory is impaired. So we can see why ADHD is associated not just with an inability to carry out tasks that involve sustained attention, but also with difficulty in completing major tasks generally. The impairment of

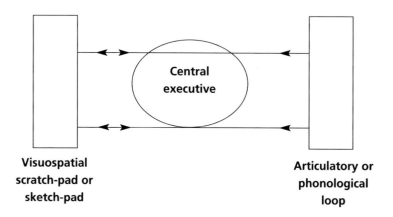

Figure 3. The working memory model of Baddeley and Hitch. (After Baddeley and Hitch, 1974. Reprinted from The Psychology of Learning & Motivation, Volume 8, Baddeley & Hitch, Working Memory, copyright 1974, with permission from Elsevier.)

executive functions also manifests as poor organizational skills, an inability to follow detailed and complicated instructions, and difficulties with any tasks that involve rearranging items or thoughts into a specific or optimum sequence.

Living within a five-second time-frame also has a particularly adverse effect on social relationships in girls. In general, non-ADHD girls appear to be more socially adept than boys and perhaps make more sophisticated use of language. Unfortunately, if you are a girl with ADHD and your timing is poor, so that, for instance, you butt in at the wrong time in conversation, then you are not going to be liked by the other girls. In fact, some researchers think that, compared with boys with ADHD, girls with ADHD may be more inattentive and disorganized.

4

What causes ADHD?

I have already mentioned some of the theories put forward to explain the cause or causes of ADHD. In this chapter I shall look in greater detail at some of the main ones, roughly in chronological order. Before doing so, however, I think it is interesting to point out that although ADHD and hyperkinetic disorder are currently diagnosed often, particularly in children and adolescents, this was not the case until the second half of the twentieth century. In retrospect, it is surprising to see that even in 1957 the main textbook on child psychiatry (the famous, to psychiatrists, third edition of Professor Leo Kanner's textbook) did not contain any reference to hyperactivity as a diagnosis. So, while reading about the following theories, it is helpful to bear in mind just how recent ADHD is as a separate diagnostic 'label'.

Written descriptions before the twentieth century

For the sake of historical completeness, I want to include two written descriptions of a childhood disorder that sound remarkably like modern-day ADHD.

The Babylonian Talmud

According to a letter published in the medical journal *Pediatrics* in 1999 by the American Dr Simon Auster (of Uniformed Services University of the Health Sciences, in Bethesda, Maryland), perhaps the earliest description of ADHD is that by Rabbi Pereda in *The Babylonian Talmud*, which makes up part of the Oral Torah of traditional orthodox Judaism. Rabbi Pereda lived in the third and fourth centuries of the Common (or Christian) Era, some one thousand seven hundred years ago. He gave a good description of the inattention and inability to concentrate on the task in hand that we now associate with ADHD:

> R[abbi] Pereda had a pupil whom he taught his lesson four hundred times before the latter could master it. On a certain day having been requested to attend to a religious matter he taught him as usual but the pupil could not master the subject. 'What', the Master asked, 'is the matter today?' 'From the moment', the other replied, 'the Master was told that there was a religious matter to be attended to I could not concentrate my thoughts, for at every moment I imagined, Now the Master will get up or Now the Master will get up.' 'Give me your attention', the Master said, 'and I will teach you again', and so he taught him another four hundred times. (Erubin (or Eiruvin) 54b, 1938 English translation.)

The Babylonian Talmud goes on to relate that Rabbi Pereda was given a choice of blessings for persevering with teaching his inattentive pupil:

> 'Do you prefer that four hundred years shall be added to your life or that you and your generations shall be privileged to have a share in the world to come? – 'That', he replied, 'I and my generations shall be privileged to have a share in the world to come.' 'Give him both', said the Holy One, blessed be He.

(Erubin (or Eiruvin) 54b, 1938 English translation.)

The story of Fidgety Philip
Fidgety Philip was one of ten stories penned by Dr Heinrich Hoffmann in his book *Der Struwwelpeter*, known in English

as *Slovenly* or *Shockheaded Peter*. A medical doctor who worked in psychiatry and lived from 1809 to 1894, Dr Hoffman wrote *Der Struwwelpeter* in 1844 for his then three-year-old son Carl Philipp. A version of the book was published in 1845, initially under the pseudonym Reimerich Kinderlieb. The story of Fidgety Philip first appeared in published form in the second edition of this book the following year. It is generally recognized as being the earliest published description, in modern times, of a child, albeit fictional, with the symptoms of ADHD. The book was copiously illustrated, making it even more fascinating to children.

In the English translation of this short story many of the modern diagnostic features of ADHD are described, including inattention, hyperactivity and impulsivity.

'Let me see if Philip can
Be a little gentleman;
Let me see if he is able
To sit still for once at the table.'
Thus spoke, in earnest tone,
The Papa to his son;
And Mama looked very grave
To see Philip so misbehave.
But Philip he did not mind
His father who was so kind.
He wriggled
And giggled,
And then, I declare,
Swung backwards and forwards
And tilted up his chair,
Just like any rocking horse; –
'Philip! I am getting cross!'
See the naughty, restless child,
Growing still more rude and wild,
Till his chair falls over quite.
Philip screams with all his might,

Catches at the cloth, but then
That makes matters worse again.
Down upon the ground they fall,
Glasses, bread, knives, forks and all.
How Mama did fret and frown,
When she saw them tumbling down!
And Papa made such a face!
Philip is in sad disgrace.

Where is Philip? Where is he?
Fairly cover'd up, you see!
Cloth and all are lying on him;
He has pull'd down all upon him!
What a terrible to-do!
Dishes, glasses, snapt in two!
Here a knife, and there fork!
Philip, this is naughty work.
Table all so bare, and ah!
Poor Papa and poor Mama
Look quite cross, and wonder how
They shall make their dinner now.

The last verse shows how the family is affected by a child with ADHD.

The story of Fidgety Philip was reproduced in the medical journal *The Lancet* in 1904. (Some authors therefore mistakenly take 1904 to be the date when this first modern account of ADHD or ADD was published.) A recent review of this story by Johannes Thome and Kerrin Jacobs that appeared in the journal *European Psychiatry* in 2004 commented as follows.

It is astonishing how clearly the typical symptoms of ADHD are depicted in Hoffmann's book. For the physician and practitioner, a few strokes of the brush and a few verses were sufficient to paint the typical picture of a child suffering from ADHD and his family. (Reproduced from Thorne and Jacobs (2004) with permission from the publishers, Elsevier.)

Mental explosivenss

In 1899, the physician Sir Thomas Smith Clouston described overexcitability or 'simple hyperexcitability' and 'mental explosiveness' in a series of 'neurotic' children. He suggested that this hyperexcitability was caused by 'undue brain reactiveness to mental and emotional stimuli', with an 'explosive' condition of the nerve cells (neurones) of the higher cerebral cortex, similar to what is believed to occur in epilepsy.

The treatment suggested for this childhood mental explosiveness was a combination of bromides (which are salts of bromine), a good diet, fresh air, and what he termed suitable amusement, companionship and employment. One of the problems with bromide treatment is that it can cause a form of poisoning known as bromism. This can lead to psychiatric symptoms, such as a lack of normal social inhibition, self-neglect, tiredness, sluggishness, impaired attention, impaired concentration, impaired memory, irritability and depression. Since some of these symptoms are, ironically, found in ADHD, it is theoretically possible that some of the children with mental explosiveness could have exhibited yet more symptoms of this condition as a result of their treatment. Other effects of bromism include neurological changes, such as headaches, slurred speech and difficulty walking, and a characteristic skin change, known as bromoderma.

Defect of moral control

In modern times, the first proper description of hyperactivity is considered to have been made by the great British paediatrician Professor Sir George Frederick Still, who lived from 1867 to 1941. He became the first professor of childhood medicine at King's College, in London, England. In a series of lectures delivered at the Royal College of Physicians in 1902, Still described a series of 20 children suffering from marked restlessness, 'an abnormal incapacity for sustained attention' and inappropriate behaviour. The children generally performed poorly at school in spite of being of normal intelligence, and the disorder was said often to be evident within the first few years of starting school. Boys were noted to suffer from this condition more than girls. These lectures were published as a series of three articles under the title 'Some abnormal psychical conditions in children' in the well-respected medical journal the *Lancet* in the same year (1902).

The cause of this disorder, according to Still, was a 'defect of moral control', with a wish on the part of the affected children for immediate gratification without regard for others or for their own long-term future. In line with the ideas of natural selection through survival of the fittest, popularized by Charles Darwin in his 1859 classic tome on evolution, *On the Origin of Species*, Frederick Still argued that moral control was the highest and most recent product of mental evolution. Being such a recent result of human evolution, moral control was also therefore vulnerable to being lost or failing to develop, according to Still.

Professor Sir Frederick Still found that many of the children who suffered from this disorder actually came from families in which there was a good standard of child-rearing. He therefore went on to modify his hypothesis and suggest that the 'defect of moral control' was the result of a 'morbid physical condition'. In turn, the putative 'morbid physical condition' was said to have been caused by heredity, a birth injury or a later injury.

In due course, children with the disorder were divided into three subgroups:

- Those with evidence of brain damage

- Those who had suffered from certain diseases and/or injuries which would normally be associated with brain damage, but in whom no such damage could be shown to exist

- Those whose behaviour was hyperactive but where the reason for this was not known.

In turn, historically these subgroups gave rise to the following three diagnostic categories:

- (Minimal) brain damage

- Minimal brain dysfunction

- Hyperactivity.

Although these terms originally referred to separate subgroups of this newly identified disorder, confusion soon set in, and each of the three terms was often used as the name of the overall disorder. As I mentioned in chapter 3, the term minimal brain damage was used during the first half of the twentieth century, gradually being replaced by minimal brain dysfunction and then hyperactivity of children (in DSM-I) by 1952.

Professor Still was knighted in 1937.

Germ corruption

During the first half of the twentieth century a different theory gained ground in some scientific circles. This was the notion that the 'the defect of moral control' thought to underlie ADHD symptoms was the result of inherited 'germ corruption'. This was particularly favoured by adherents of the eugenics movement. One prominent member of this movement was the British physician Alfred Frank Tredgold, who served on the English Royal Commission on Mental Deficiency. He described several cases of childhood hyperactivity in his book *Mental Deficiency (Amentia)*, which was first published in 1908, and said to be the first description of children suffering from 'minimal brain damage'.

In the eighth edition of his textbook, published in 1952, Tredgold described those thought to have a mental defect but who were not severely intellectually impaired as being 'feebleminded', and as suffering from deficiencies in:

- Common sense

- Judgement

- The inhibition of primitive instincts, and

- 'Active attention'.

As a consequence, patients were said to lack the ability to control, co-ordinate and adapt their conduct to the requirements of their surroundings.

Tredgold believed that the slum environments from which many of the hyperactive 'high-grade feebleminded' children hailed were usually the result rather than the cause of their 'pronounced morbid inheritance'. Some of the terms used by Tredgold to describe the inherited brain defect that gave rise to hyperactivity included:

- Germ corruption

- Blastophoria

- Neuropathic diathesis, and

- Psychopathic diathesis.

Alfred Tredgold complained that, rather than following the example of 'Ancient Eugenics', as in the case of the ancient Spartans, and allowing the unfit to die at or soon after birth, modern science was being used 'to keep alight the feeble flame of life in the baseborn child of a degenerate parent' (*Eugenics and the Future Progress of Man*). Consistent with these views, Tredgold advocated the sterilization of the 'mentally deficient'.

Encephalitis lethargica

Another cause that was advanced for ADHD-like features was encephalitis lethargica.

Towards the end of the First World War, there was a worldwide influenza pandemic of horrific proportions that killed many millions of people. Starting in 1917, some of the survivors of this pandemic developed a terrible condition in which they became essentially mute and hardly able to move, as if they were living statues. (The condition often started with headaches, malaise, lethargy, insomnia and strange eye movements.) Most of those affected by this condition, known as encephalitis lethargica or von Economo encephalitis, were institutionalized for life; some of the long-term sufferers in an institution in New York were brilliantly described by Dr Oliver Sacks in his book *Awakenings*.

Some children and adolescents suffered from a post-encephalitic syndrome, known as 'post-encephalitic behaviour disorder', in which their behaviour was disturbed. Symptoms included hyperactivity, impulsivity, poor coordination, aggression, learning disability, changes in personality, and sometimes also reduced attention. Because obvious brain disease could not generally be found, it was assumed that there must be 'minimal' brain damage. Therefore, the terms 'minimal brain disease' and then 'minimal brain dysfunction' were used to describe children and adolescents with the symptoms and signs we now associate with ADHD.

As the epidemic of encephalitis lethargica followed closely on the influenza pandemic (caused by a virus), it was naturally assumed by some scientists that if it were indeed a genuine neurological illness it too was caused by a virus. (There were some psychiatrists who attributed this condition to purely psychosomatic or 'hysterical' causes.) However, though there were certainly features of the condition that pointed to an infection, to date, no genetic material of any influenza virus or indeed any virus at all has been found in the post mortem (autopsy) brains of affected patients.

Meanwhile, since the end of the First World War right up to the present day, more people have developed encephalitis lethargica although it is now far less common. In 2004, Dr Russell Dale, working at the Institute of Child Health at Great Ormond Street Hospital, London, published a paper in the journal *Brain* in which he and his colleagues showed evidence that patients who had developed encephalitis lethargica more recently had been infected not by a virus but by a bacterium, namely the *Streptococcus*. In fact, most patients with the illness have had a (Strep) sore throat before the start of their symptoms. An increasing number of neuropsychiatric disorders that follow streptococcal infection have now been found to be associated with antibodies acting against two important centres, or nuclei, of grey matter deep inside the brain called the basal ganglia (Martino and Giovannoni, 2004). Since the basal ganglia are involved in the control of movement, it is interesting to speculate that antibodies acting against the basal ganglia, formed as a result of a Streptococcal infection, might be responsible for the hyperactivity seen in ADHD. At the time of writing, however, there is little evidence to support this hypothesis.

Hyperkinetic disease

During the first half of the 1930s, Dr Kramer-Pollnow described a series of 15 children suffering from a syndrome of unusual restlessness, distractibility and speech disorder. The restlessness had often started suddenly, typically at the age of three or four years, and was often followed by an epileptic fit. The syndrome was named 'hyperkinetische Erkrankung' (or 'hyperkinetic disease') by Kramer-Pollnow. The cause was not known.

'Organic driveness'

In 1934, Eugen Kahn and Louis H. Cohen published an influential paper in the *New England Journal of Medicine* in which they described hyperactive (and intelligent) children and adults. These patients showed behaviour that had the following characteristics:

- 'Choreiform' or tic-like movements. Choreiform movements are writhing dance-like movements, seen for example in Huntington's disease (also known for this reason as Huntington's chorea). Tics are repeated irregular movements involving a particular group of muscles. (Tics are also seen in Huntington's disease, for example)

- Extreme difficulty in staying quiet or still

- Clumsy movements

- An 'explosive' quality to voluntary movement.

Kahn and Cohen suggested that these four symptoms were related to the functioning of the part of the brain known as the brain stem. This is a relatively primitive part of the brain, which directly connects, below, with the spinal cord, as shown in Figure 4. Furthermore, Kahn and Cohen noted that there had been cases of changes in personality and behaviour that were related to encephalitis lethargica affecting the brain stem. Therefore, these authors proposed that the hyperactivity syndrome they had identified was caused by an organic disorder affecting the brain stem. They termed this cause of hyperactivity 'organic driveness' and suggested it could occur 'from birth, either as the consequence of a prenatal encephalopathy or injury or of birth injury, or as a constitutional variant'.

This theory did not stand the test of time. These days, researchers are more likely to think that the cerebral cortex is more important than the brain stem in causing ADHD. This was even pointed out at the time of publication of Kahn & Cohen's paper in 1934.

Neurotransmitter changes in the brain

In these days of high-resolution MRI (magnetic resonance imaging) scanners, it is easy to forget how difficult it was to obtain images of the brain in living patients before the 1970s. In that decade Sir Godfrey Newbold Housfield invented computerized axial tomography (CAT or CT scanning), and since then MRI has been added to the technologies available to doctors wanting to obtain high-quality images of the functioning brain.

In late 1895, the German professor of physics, Wilhelm Conrad Roentgen (1845 to 1923) formally announced his discovery of

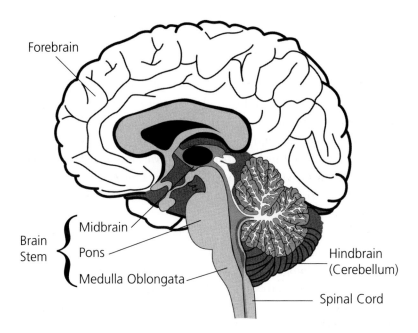

Figure 4. Section through the brain showing the brain stem.

X-rays. During his report to the Wurzburg Physical-Medical Society on 28th December 1895, Roentgen showed an X-ray image of one of his wife's hands. This famous image, taken on 22nd December of that year, showed many of the bones in her hand, and also a dark shadow on one of her fingers, which I imagine was a ring.

X-rays soon entered medical practice. They were very useful for diagnosing bone fractures and lung diseases, to give just two examples. When it came to X-rays of the head, however, it soon became apparent that the brain did not show up. This technique was not therefore much used in studying brain disorders. (Having said that, there are exceptions. With two of my colleagues, I published a skull X-ray of a 36-year-old man suffering from thoughts of being persecuted. The X-ray of his skull does not show up his brain at all. It does, however, show a three-inch masonry nail in his brain. The patient had held the nail against a wall and head-butted its point until he had driven it fully into his forehead. The interested reader can see the X-ray in the paper by Puri, El-Dosoky and Barrett, 1994, or in the *Textbook of Psychiatry* by Puri, Laking and Treasaden.)

Most people know that the human heart has four chambers, the two largest of which are known as ventricles. Perhaps less well known is that the human brain also contains four chambers; in this case all four are known as ventricles. Figure 5 shows these. The two largest are the left and right lateral ventricles, which are each connected to the third ventricle. In turn, the third ventricle is connected, via the cerebral aqueduct, to the fourth ventricle. In turn, the fourth ventricle of the brain is connected to the central canal of the spinal cord.

Normally, the ventricles are filled with cerebrospinal fluid. Since the ventricles are connected to the central canal of the spinal cord, this canal usually also contains cerebrospinal fluid. This is why it is possible for doctors to obtain a sample of cerebrospinal fluid by carrying out a 'spinal tap' or lumbar puncture.

In 1918, Walter Dandy discovered that it was possible to obtain X-ray images of the ventricles of the brain, and some adjacent brain structures, by replacing the cerebrospinal fluid with air. Professor Walter Edward Dandy, who lived from 1886 to 1946, was one of the most outstanding neurosurgeons of the first half of the twentieth century. He was the second Professor of Neurological Surgery at Johns Hopkins Hospital in Baltimore, Maryland, succeeding the famous Professor Harvey Cushing. The method that Walter Dandy first used involved pumping air directly into the ventricles of the brain either through holes that were drilled in the skull, or by entering through a fontanelle (a soft part of the skull between bones that have not yet fused in a baby). This highly invasive technique was soon replaced by what was essentially the reverse of a lumbar puncture (spinal tap): cerebrospinal fluid would be removed through a needle inserted into the central canal of the spinal cord at the level of the lumbar spine, and replaced by air. If the patient was upright, the air would rise up through the central canal of the spinal cord to fill the ventricles of the brain. The patient's head could then be X-rayed. This technique was named 'ventriculography' by Dandy, but came to be better known in medical circles by the name given to it by Dr Bingel in Germany, namely 'pneumoencephalography', or air encephalography. Pneumoencephalography was widely used during much of the twentieth century to take images of the brain, until the advent of, first, CT scanners (also known as EMI or CAT scanners) and then MRI scanners.

For the next part of our story, we have to move from the Johns Hopkins Hospital in Baltimore, Maryland, to the Emma Pendleton Bradley Home (now known as Bradley Hospital) in East Providence, Rhode Island. An only child, Emma Pendleton Bradley was born in 1880 to George Lathrop Bradley, who was a very wealthy mining engineer, and his wife. Sadly, Emma developed encephalitis (inflammation of the brain, usually caused by an infection) during her

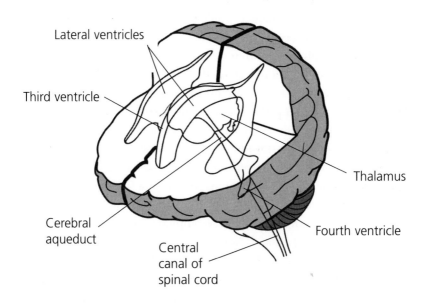

Figure 5. The four venticles of the human brain. These consist of the two large lateral ventricles, the third ventricle (under the left lateral ventricle) and the fourth ventricle.

childhood, and was left with behavioural problems, cerebral palsy and epilepsy. Emma died in 1907, at the age of twenty-seven. The previous year, her father died. In his will, he left funds to open a home for poor children who were suffering from illnesses similar to Emma's, and to carry out research into such disorders. The home was to be built after the death of Emma's mother, which occurred in 1919. The Emma Pendleton Bradley Home was opened in 1931. The second superintendent and medical director, appointed in 1932, was Dr Charles Bradley. Charles shared the same surname as the founder because George Lathrop Bradley was Charles' great-uncle.

Dr Charles Bradley, who was born in 1902, had studied paediatrics and neurology, and joined the Emma Pendleton Bradley Home after completing a residency at Babies Hospital in New York. He carried out extensive neurological testing of the children with ADHD-like features referred to the Emma Pendleton Bradley Home, including pneumoencephalography. In fact, he invented a chair specifically designed to speed up the performance of pneumoencephalography in children.

An unsurprising side-effect of draining out cerebrospinal fluid from the ventricles of the brain and replacing it with air is that the person undergoing this procedure may suffer from headaches. During the 1930s, amphetamines (or amfetamines) were available for prescription as stimulants to adults in the United States. Dr Charles Bradley actually started prescribing amphetamine, under the trade name Benzedrine, to children who were suffering from headaches following the invasive procedure of pneumoencephalography. (Benzedrine is actually amphetamine sulphate, or more officially, the Recommended International Non-proprietary Name is amfetamine sulfate.) He reasoned that, being a potent stimulant drug, Benzedrine/amphetamine would stimulate the brain to produce more cerebrospinal fluid after the pneumoencephalography procedure was over. In turn, this would help ease the painful headaches.

(For those interested in chemical structures, Figure 6 shows a molecule of Benzedrine/amphetamine. This cannot be shown in a 2-dimensional diagam, but in the same way that gloves come in pairs, so amphetamine has two versions, a right-hand and a left-hand type. Benzedrine consists of both the right-hand version (known as dextroamphetamine, *d*-amphetamine, dextroamfetamine

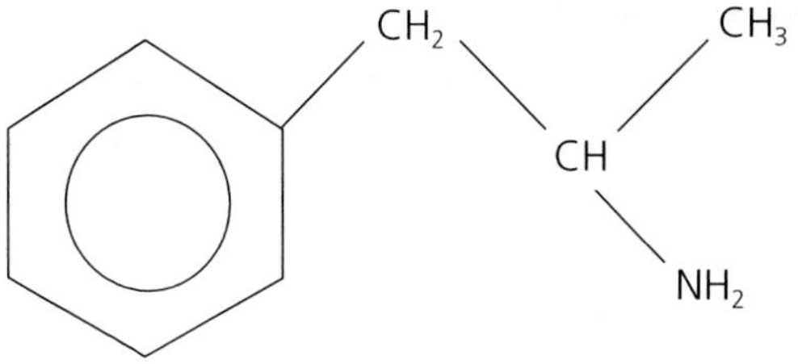

Figure 6. Benzedrine (amphetamine).

or *d*-amfetamine) and the left-hand version (levoamphetamine, *l*-amphetamine, levoamfetamine or *l*-amfetamine).)

Charles Bradley was wrong. The Benzedrine did not particularly help the children's headaches. However, unexpectedly, their teachers noticed that some of the hyperactive children appeared to find it easier to sit still and concentrate in class. In fact, it is said that some of the children started to refer to their Benzedrine/amphetamine treatment as 'arithmetic pills' because of the benefits to their school work. As a result, he carried out a small study in 30 children.

In 1937, Dr Charles Bradley published a paper in the *American Journal of Psychiatry*, called 'The behavior of children receiving Benzedrine'. In this paper he reported that out of 30 children with behavioural problems, 14 had shown a 'spectacular change in behavior' and 'remarkably improved school performance'. To quote more fully, Bradley stated that:

Possibly the most striking change in behavior during the week of Benzedrine therapy occurred in the school activities of many of these patients…There appeared a definite 'drive' to accomplish as much as possible during the school period, and often to spend extra time completing additional work. Speed of comprehension and accuracy of performance were increased in most cases…It appeared promptly on the first day Benzedrine was given and disappeared on the first day it was discontinued.

This then, is the real foundation for the use of powerful psychostimulants, including amphetamine and amphetamine-like drugs, in children with ADHD. Note that it was not the case that a scientifically sound hypothesis was formulated on the basis of the clinical features of ADHD, and that a systematic treatment approach was then tried on this firm foundation. On the contrary, a powerful stimulant used in adults in the 1930s, namely amphetamine, was given to hyperactive children who suffered headaches as a result of having cerebrospinal fluid drained from their brains, and, purely by chance it was found that the amphetamine helped their behaviour. (A note on spelling is appropriate here. The traditional spelling amphetamine, as used in much of the English-speaking world, even the United States of America, has changed in the United Kingdom in respect of its use as a pharmacological agent. As a result of European Union law, British Approved Names have had to be changed to harmonize them with the Recommended International Non-proprietary Names. This means that, in medical texts dealing with amphetamines as prescription drugs, the spelling has been changed to amfetamines. For the purposes of this book, I have decided to continue to use the traditional spelling. In making this decision, I have tried not to be influenced too much by my long-standing views on the European Union, which could easily fill another book!)

In due course, a number of different powerful psychostimulant drugs were developed and marketed for the growing problem of childhood ADHD. These included Ritalin, Dexedrine and Cylert. They became the drugs of first choice and some, such as Ritalin, achieved enormous sales. There were some problems, however.

One major problem was that, as would be expected, prescribing powerful psychostimulants to children causes many major unwanted side-effects. After all, it is not without good reason that most responsible governments ban the recreational use of amphetamines, cocaine, and other psychostimulants in their countries. I shall look at these side-effects in detail in Chapter 6.

Another problem was more philosophical, and concerned the lack of any scientific rationale for this newly found first-line 'treatment' for ADHD. If a child is already overactive, how could it make sense to give them a stimulant; and not just a mild stimulant but a powerful psychostimulant whose parent compound is deemed too dangerous even for non-ADHD adults to use? Companies profiting from the increasing sales of such drugs were willing to spend large sums to sponsor research activities by psychiatrists who would seek some scientific rationale for this serendipitous treatment. This has spawned a large body of research findings, particularly in the fields of neurotransmitters (the chemical messengers that act between brain cells), and, more recently, brain imaging. A whole edifice of theories has been constructed to support various neurotransmitter/brain imaging models that suggest that the right way to treat ADHD is with stimulant medication.

I shall therefore turn now to the action of psychostimulants on neurotransmission. This section is complicated and includes a fair amount of neuroanatomy. If you find yourself getting lost do just fast-forward to the summary on pages 74–75.

Psychostimulants and neurotransmission

The main way in which brain cells (or neurones) in humans communicate is by means of chemicals known as neurotransmitters. These include substances such as dopamine, noradrenaline (also known as norepinephrine), serotonin (also known as 5-hydroxytrypt-amine, or 5-HT for short), gamma-amino butyric acid (or GABA for short) and glutamate (or glutamic acid). Under the microscope, you can see that individual neurones do not make direct contact with each other in the brain. This has been likened to the way in which the finger of Adam and the finger of the Almighty do not quite meet in Michelangelo's fresco of the Creation of Adam, in the Sistine Chapel in the Vatican. The tiny gap between brain cells is known as the synaptic cleft. For a signal to pass from one brain cell (the presynaptic neurone) to an adjoining neurone (the postsynaptic neurone), a neurotransmitter leaves the first brain cell and has to cross the synaptic cleft and attach to a receptor on the surface of the postsynaptic neurone. This whole process is called neurotransmission.

There are a number of different neurotransmitters in the brain. Both the right-handed amphetamine (dextroamphetamine or *d*-amphetamine) in Benzedrine and a psychostimulant commonly used in ADHD, namely methylphenidate (proprietary name, Ritalin), act mainly on one particular neurotransmitter, dopamine. They release this neurotransmitter into the synaptic cleft, and possibly also stop it being carried away, as shown in Figure 7.

We know that there is an important pathway containing dopamine brain cells which starts from an ancient region deep in the brain stem (the ventral tegmental area) and reaches forward to 'innervate' (that is, send nerve cell branches to) parts of the frontal lobe and more ancient limbic system. Parts of the frontal lobes that are innervated include the 'dorsolateral prefrontal cortex'. This region, it is believed, may contain some of our 'free will' brain circuits. The limbic system is involved in processing the sense of smell, in emotions, in learning and in memory. The dopamine pathway from the ventral tegmental area to the limbic system also

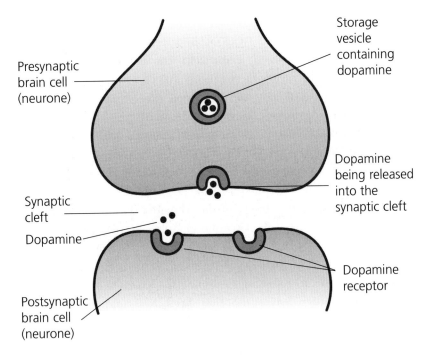

Figure 7. Dopamine neurotransmission.

innervates part of the inner frontal lobes (the medial prefrontal cortex); these regions are called the mesocortical region (or area) and the pathway is referred to as the mesocortical system. This is shown diagrammatically in Figure 8.

Textbooks now tend to tell us a rather different story. They generally state that this dopamine pathway (from the ventral tegmental area to the mesocortical and dorsolateral prefrontal cortical regions) may mediate functions such as attention, arousal and concentration. The evidence for this is not always given, but if it is, will often include reference to work with animals, particularly rodents. Modern textbooks then go on to recommend certain psychostimulants for the treatment of ADHD because of their alleged beneficial action on this dopamine pathway. The argument goes something like this:

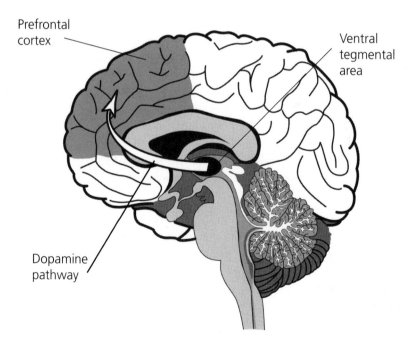

Figure 8. The dopamine pathway from the ventral tegmental area (in the brain stem) to the prefrontal cortex (in the frontal lobes).

- Amphetamine is serendipitously found (by Charles Bradley) to help improve attention, arousal and concentration in children with ADHD

- Amphetamine improves dopamine neurotransmission

- A key dopamine brain pathway passes from the ventral tegmental area of the brain stem to the mesocortical and dorsolateral prefrontal cortical regions

- Therefore this dopamine pathway is involved in the functions of attention, arousal and concentration. (Some rodent work is produced to back up this claim.)

- Since this dopamine pathway is involved in the functions of attention, arousal and concentration, it would make sense to use drugs that stimulate this pathway to treat ADHD

- Amphetamine (particularly dextroamphetamine or *d*-amphetamine) and methylphenidate (e.g. Ritalin) stimulate this dopamine pathway

- Therefore, there is good scientific justification for using amphetamine, methylphenidate, and other similar powerful psychostimulants to treat ADHD. The improvement seen in ADHD with these drugs is evidence that the scientific foundation must be right.

This may appear to be rather a circular argument. To be fair to its advocates, I should point out that many leading psychiatrists point to two further factors that appear to support it. First, it has been suggested that patients with ADHD, when they become adults, 'self-medicate' with psychostimulants, suggesting that perhaps they need psychostimulants. Second, genes related to dopamine neurotransmission have been found to be abnormal in ADHD. Let us examine each of these further pieces of evidence in turn.

The need for psychostimulants

It is certainly true that adult (and adolescent) patients with ADHD smoke more than would be expected in the general population. For example, in 1995, Pomerleau and colleagues, of the Behavioral Medicine Program of the University of Michigan Department of Psychiatry, in Ann Arbor, published a paper in the *Journal of Substance Abuse* investigating the smoking habits of 71 adult patients with ADHD. Whereas almost 41% of the adults with ADHD were current smokers, the comparable figure for the general population in 1991, unselected for ADHD, was just under 26%. They also examined the percentages of people who had ever smoked who were currently ex-smokers; this was termed the 'quit ratio'. Whereas the quit ratio for the ADHD adults was 29%, it was much higher, at 48.5%, in the general population.

In another study published in 1988 in the journal *Biological Psychiatry*, by Joseph Biederman and colleagues from the Pediatric Psychopharmacology Clinic of Massachusetts General Hospital, Boston, 239 adults with ADHD were compared with 268 non-ADHD healthy adults. They found that the adults with ADHD were far more likely to abuse psychoactive substances (such as alcohol and illicit drugs) than were the non-ADHD adults. In fact, 55% of the ADHD group had engaged in substance abuse at some time in their lives, compared with only 27% of the non-ADHD (control) group. In clinical practice, it appears that one particularly common drug of abuse in ADHD is cannabis; there is also a fair amount of alcohol abuse as well.

So there is good evidence for a high rate of psychostimulant abuse in adults (and adolescents) with ADHD. But does this necessarily imply that ADHD subjects in some way 'require' psychostimulants and should be prescribed these? For a more considered answer, we need to carry out a deeper examination of one of the functions of dopamine.

There is ample evidence that dopamine is a neurotransmitter that has a key involvement in the perception of pleasure. We, and other mammals, have several 'pleasure centres' in our brains, and dopamine appears to be involved as a major neurotransmitter in each one. An example of just how powerfully addictive is the release of dopamine in a brain pleasure centre is shown by an experiment that was first carried out in the 1950s. In 1954, James Olds and Peter Milner published a paper in the *Journal of Comparative and Physiological Psychology* in which they placed an electrode deep inside the brain of a rat (actually inside the septal area or region of the hypothalamus). The experimental arrangement was such that every time the rat pressed on a small lever, the electrode was stimulated. In turn this led to the release of dopamine in the pleasure centre and, presumably, to a sensation of pleasure. A typical rat in such an experiment will keep pressing the lever repeatedly. Sometimes, if it has the energy, it may press the lever up to four thousand times per hour – more than once every second! In fact, rats in such experiments have been found to prefer pressing the lever to other activities – even activities important to the maintenance of health such as eating and drinking water. In some subsequent experiments dehydrated and starving rodents have actually died because of their preference for stimulating dopamine release in a brain pleasure centre. This puts in context the addictive potential in humans of dopamine-releasing psychostimulants such as amphetamine and methylphenidate.

Some of these pleasure centres form part of the brain reward system in humans (and other mammals). In ADHD, patients have an abnormality of their brain reward system. They make decisions that maximize the immediate reward, while paying scant attention to the medium- to long-term. Take two eight-year-old children and give them a choice. They can either have one chocolate bar right now, or, if they wait 30 seconds they can have two chocolate bars. A normal child without ADHD is more likely than not to choose the second option. But a child with ADHD is likely to take the first option. Children with ADHD act as if they are living within a five-second time-frame. Such an abnormality of the brain reward system (christened 'reward deficiency syndrome' by Ken Blum of the Department of Pharmacology at the University of Texas Health Science Center in San Antonio) is associated with abnormal functioning of the dopamine system in the brain (particularly the dopamine D_2 receptor). In addition to ADHD, reward deficiency syndrome has also been implicated in cases of addiction and pathological gambling. It is argued that the deficiency of internal (brain) rewards may drive the person to 'self-medicate' by seeking substances (alcohol, tobacco, illicit drugs) or engaging in behaviours (such as over-eating, gambling or sexually promiscuous activity) that release dopamine in the pleasure centres of the brain. Just as we do not feel it is right to pander to the hedonistic desires of the drug addict or compulsive gambler, perhaps it is not right to use dopamine-stimulating psychostimulants as a first-line treatment in ADHD.

Abnormal genes related to dopamine neurotransmission

With regard to genes related to dopamine neurotransmission, it is certainly true that some abnormalities have been found in ADHD. At the time of writing, two such genes in particular have been implicated. Look again at Figure 7. The dopamine receptor on the postsynaptic brain cell is made of a protein. As with all proteins, the genetic code for making it is found in genes in the DNA. There are several different types of dopamine receptor proteins. One, the D_2 receptor, has just been mentioned. It turns out that there is evidence that a variant for the D_4 receptor gene sometimes occurs in ADHD. (See, for example, Durston and colleagues, 2005; or Leung and colleagues, 2005.) (An abbreviation commonly used for the dopamine D_4 receptor is DRD4.)

Another gene abnormality in ADHD relates to a protein which helps transport dopamine, called dopamine transporter or DAT1 (or sometimes SLC6A3). Dopamine transporter terminates the action of dopamine at the synapse (see Figure 7) by carrying dopamine back into the presynaptic brain cell. In fact, amphetamine and methylphenidate (and cocaine, for that matter) target this protein: blocking the action of dopamine transporter is one of the ways in which these drugs increase the amount of dopamine in the synaptic cleft. Again, a variant for the dopamine transporter gene also sometimes occurs in ADHD. (See, for example, Cornish and colleagues, 2005; or Durston and colleagues, 2005.)

Genetic studies looking at twins and siblings indicate that there is an important genetic component to ADHD, but the variations in the dopamine-related DRD4 and DAT1 genes just mentioned appear to account for only a tiny fraction of this genetic component. (The other genetic factors involved are not yet understood.) To quantify this, we need to remind ourselves of the meaning of the term odds. (If you regularly bet on sporting events, you will likely already be familiar with this.) The odds of an event occurring is simply the ratio of the chances of that event occurring to the chances that it does not occur. Taking this one step further, in the present context of ADHD, the odds ratio is the ratio of the odds of having ADHD in one group to the odds of having it in another (control) group. So, if we have a putative gene abnormality associated with ADHD, we might suppose that the odds ratio will be fairly large. This is just not so in the cases of the dopamine-related DRD4 and DAT1 genes. The odds ratio associated with the DRD4 abnormality is not even two – in fact around 1.44. So if you have two groups of children, the first with the DRD4 gene change and the other without, then the odds of having ADHD in the first group is only 1.44 times the odds of having it in the second group. For the DAT1 gene change, the odds ratio falls even further to a miserly 1.13.

There are now screening tests available for the DRD4 gene. Screening costs around £20 or $40 (US); it is not currently useful and parents should not waste their money on it.

So to summarize:

- Some brain pathways use the chemical dopamine for communication between brain cells

- Some of the psychostimulants used to treat ADHD (such as Benzedrine in the past and methylphenidate or Ritalin these days) act on dopamine

- This has led to a circular argument about the role of dopamine and psychostimulants in ADHD

- It is true that ADHD patients have a greater tendency to 'self-medicate', especially as adults. But this does not prove that they need psychostimulants. The addictive substances or behaviours can release dopamine in key 'reward' regions of the brain, and this goes to show just how strong the addictive potential of psychostimulants can be

- It is also true that genes relating to dopamine have been found to be abnormal in ADHD patients. However, these abnormalities account for only a tiny fraction of the total genetic component to ADHD.

In contrast to psychostimulant therapy, in the next chapter I shall describe an approach to the treatment of ADHD that is based on carefully thought out, strong scientific and clinical foundations. This new treatment method also has the advantage of being entirely natural.

5

How and why fatty acids can help

If you are not familiar with the concepts of human biology, you will find this chapter the most difficult in the book. It relates to the area of research in which I have been working for many years – the role played by fatty acids in health and disease. It is this work that has led me to the conclusion that many conditions, including ADHD, result from fatty acid deficiencies. So that you can understand exactly what fatty acids are and why they are fundamental to ADHD I have included quite a lot of cell biology, I hope in a form that you will be able to follow. Fatty acids are essential constituents of every living cell in the human body so I will start with cells and cell membranes.

What are fatty acids?

Cell membranes

All our organs are made of tissues, which in turn are made of cells. Cells are the structural and functional units of all living organisms, including humans. There are many different types of cell in our organs. For example, in the brain there are neurones (brain cells) and glial cells. In the blood there are red blood cells and white blood cells. A diagram of a typical human cell, in section, is shown in Figure 9.

All our living cells have a boundary double-layer called the cell membrane, as shown in Figure 9. Similar double-layered membranes also surround certain structures inside cells, called organelles. Examples of organelles include the mitochondria (which are the powerhouses of the cell) and the nucleus (which contains the genetic information of the cell in the form of DNA or deoxyribonucleic acid). The double-layered membrane around the nucleus is called the nuclear envelope.

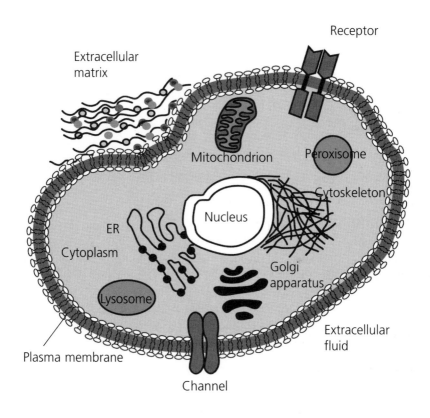

Figure 9. A typical human cell. 'ER' is endoplasmic reticulum. The receptors and channels on the outside of the cell are proteins lying within the cell membrane.

In Figure 9 you can see neurotransmitter receptors in the outer cell membrane. These receptors are protein molecules. A normal cell membrane is fluid – the protein receptors in the cell membrane have considerable freedom of movement within the two-layered membrane. Figure 10 shows the structure of a typical cell membrane.

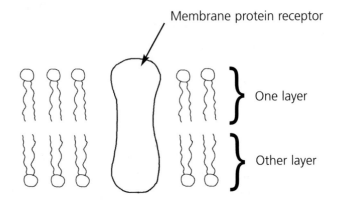

Figure 10. The structure of a typical cell membrane.

Phospholipids

Cell membranes are made of two layers of molecules called phospholipids. A close-up of one of these phospholipid molecules is shown in Figure 11.

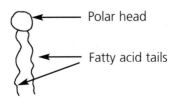

Figure 11. A close-up of a phospholipid molecule.

Each phospholipid molecule has a water-loving ('hydrophilic' or 'polar') head component. Attached to this polar head component are two tails. These tails are water-hating ('hydrophobic'). Each tail is a fatty or lipid molecule called a fatty acid. As a result of the fact that the polar head components are attracted to water whereas the fatty acid tails are water-hating, the phospholipid molecules arrange themselves in the manner shown in Figure 10. That is, they form a double-layer, in which the polar head components face outwards, towards the watery environment of the fluid outside the cell and the watery environment of the fluid (cytoplasm) inside the cell. Meanwhile, the fatty acid tails are in a stable position by lying in a fatty environment away from the more watery environments just outside and inside the cell (or organelle).

Fatty acids

Fatty acids are the water-hating fatty tails shown in Figures 10 and 11. In cell membranes, they tend to be long molecules, made up mainly of carbon and hydrogen atoms. Most of the bonds between adjacent carbon atoms in a fatty acid molecule are known as single-bonds. Occasionally, stronger double-bonds occur. For those of you with an interest in chemistry, Figure 12 shows the difference between a single-bond and a double-bond.

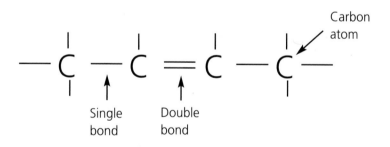

Figure 12. The difference between a single-bond and a double-bond between carbon atoms.

Fatty acids vary according to the total number of carbon atoms, the total number of double-bonds, and the positions of the double-bonds. Those fatty acids that have their first double-bond starting at the sixth carbon atom from a particular end of the molecule are known as omega-6 fatty acids. Similarly, those fatty acids that have their first double-bond starting at the third carbon atom from the same end of the molecule are known as omega-3 fatty acids. These are very important molecules. You may, for example, have come across the advice of the American Heart Association (published as *Fish Consumption, Fish Oil, Omega-3 fatty acids and Cardiovascular Heart Disease* in 2002) extolling the virtues of omega-3 fatty acids:

> Omega-3 fatty acids benefit the heart of healthy people, and those at high risk of – or who have – cardiovascular disease. ...**We recommend eating fish (particularly fatty fish) at least two times a week.** Fish is a good source of protein and doesn't have the high saturated fat that fatty meat products do. Fatty fish like mackerel, lake trout, herring, sardines, albacore tuna and salmon are high in two kinds of omega-3 fatty acids, **eicosapentaenoic acid (EPA) and docosahexaenoic acid (DHA).** (Reproduced with permission,www.americanheart.org,http://www.americanheart.org/presenter.jhtml?identifier=4632. ©2005, American Heart Association.)

As well as preventing heart disease, omega-3 fatty acids (particularly EPA) have many other health benefits. These will be described in Chapter 8.

Meanwhile, it will help us understand better the role of fatty acids in ADHD if we know a little about how the body obtains its supply of different omega-3 and omega-6 fatty acids.

How the body obtains omega-3 and omega-6 fatty acids

Figure 13 summarizes the most important omega-3 and omega-6 fatty acids and how the body makes them. Basically, the first omega-6 fatty acid at the top of the left-hand chain, named linoleic acid (LA), can be obtained from certain foodstuffs, especially vegetable oils (sunflower oil is particularly rich in LA) but cannot be made by our bodies. Once we have LA in our bodies (from food) in theory we have the chemical machinery to create all the succeeding omega-6 fatty acids below LA in the left-hand omega-6 chain. Thus, our cells can, in theory, convert LA into gamma-linolenic acid (GLA). In turn, GLA can be converted into dihomo-gamma-linolenic acid (DGLA). This in turn can be converted into arachidonic acid (AA), and so on.

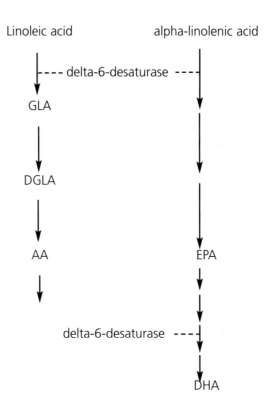

OMEGA-6 FATTY ACIDS   **OMEGA-3 FATTY ACIDS**

Linoleic acid   alpha-linolenic acid

delta-6-desaturase

GLA

DGLA

AA   EPA

delta-6-desaturase

DHA

Figure 13. Omega-3 and omega-6 fatty acids.

Similarly, on the omega-3 side, the first omega-3 fatty acid at the top of the right-hand chain, named alpha-linolenic acid (ALA), can be obtained from certain foodstuffs (for example, nuts and seeds) but cannot be made by our bodies. Once we have ALA in our bodies (from food), in theory we have the chemical machinery to create all the succeeding omega-3 fatty acids below ALA that are shown in the right-hand omega-3 chain.

Each succeeding step in the chain requires the help of a particular naturally occurring enzyme. These enzymes speed up, or 'catalyze', chemical reactions that would otherwise take far too long to be useful. As an example, consider what would happen if you were to eat a teaspoonful of ordinary white sugar (or sucrose, to give it its proper name). Assuming that you are not overweight and that you are exercising sufficiently to need some energy, then the sugar would react with oxygen (ultimately derived from the air you breathe in) and be converted into carbon dioxide gas and water, in your body. In the process of this happening, the conversion would release a fair amount of energy, which you could use, for example to walk, read or think. However, if you do not consume the sugar and just leave it lying on your table, it is highly unlikely that it will undergo any such reaction, even though it is surrounded by air that is rich in oxygen. The same reaction that occurs rapidly in the body, because of the help of enzymes, is usually excruciatingly slow at room temperature without the presence of the enzymes. The enzymes required for the omega-3 and omega-6 fatty acid conversions are the same at any given stage in Figure 13. For instance, the enzyme that helps convert the omega-6 fatty acid LA into GLA is known as delta-6-desaturase. It is this same enzyme that aids the conversion of ALA into the next omega-3 fatty acid in the omega-3 chain.

Since LA and ALA have to be provided by our diet and cannot be manufactured from scratch by our bodies, they are known as 'essential fatty acids'. The succeeding omega-3 and omega-6 fatty acids, particularly those with 20 or 22 carbon atoms, are known variously as long-chain polyunsaturated fatty acids, LC-PUFAs, highly unsaturated fatty acids, or HUFAs. These include DGLA and AA, on the omega-6 side, and eicosapentaenoic acid (EPA) and docosahexaenoic acid (DHA) on the omega-3 side.

What do omega-3 and omega-6 fatty acids do?

Structure of membranes
The omega-3 and omega-6 fatty acids have extremely important roles in maintaining the correct structure of cell membranes throughout the

body. In particular, for a membrane to function properly, it needs to have sufficient levels of the omega-6 long-chain polyunsaturated fatty acid arachidonic acid (AA), and the omega-3 long-chain polyunsaturated fatty acid docosahexaenoic acid (DHA). Without these fatty acids, instead of being fluid, cell membranes become more rigid, and this reduced flexibility is reflected in poorer or abnormal functioning of receptors that lie in the membranes. In turn, this means that communication between cells, including between brain cells, is impaired.

Eicosanoids

Even more importantly, two of the omega-6 long-chain polyunsaturated fatty acids, dihomo-gamma-linolenic acid (DGLA) and arachidonic acid (AA), and one of the omega-3 long-chain polyunsaturated fatty acids, namely eicosapentaenoic acid (EPA), act as the starting point for the manufacture, by the body, of many different vital substances, including:

- Families of prostaglandins

- Families of thromboxanes

- Families of hydroxy fatty acids, and

- Families of leukotrienes.

So important are these substances that whole textbooks have been written on individual members of each of these families. In essence, these substances, which collectively are called eicosanoids, are special types of hormones that act on nearby cells after being created, rather than being transported long distances in the body to cells and tissues that lie far away from their site of synthesis. They are involved in many processes that are important in maintaining the health and well-being of the body and in fighting disease, including:

- Blood clotting

- Regulating blood pressure

- Reproduction

- The response to disease or trauma (including inflammation responses, pain and fever), and

- The secretion of acid by the stomach.

Sleep

When there is sufficient EPA (eicosapentaenoic acid) available to the body, it can be converted into natural sleep mediators. This is one of the reasons that my patients and acquaintances enjoy such wonderful, deep, refreshing sleep when they follow my advice to take a formulation each day that contains ultra-pure EPA (that is, EPA without any DHA). (In chapter 7 I shall consider the best ways to take fatty acids.)

Effect on viruses

The omega-3 fatty acid EPA (eicosapentaenoic acid) has a particularly important role in helping the body to combat viral infections. It turns out that EPA can actually kill viruses in the body, without harming us in the process. It does this in at least two ways.

First, EPA is itself directly 'viricidal'. In other words, if you add small amounts of EPA solution to harmful viruses (such as the Epstein Barr virus that causes glandular fever), then the EPA actually kills the virus.

Second, EPA is also indirectly viricidal. After being acted on by two sets of enzymes, known as COX (cyclo-oxygenase) and LOX (lipo-oxygenase), EPA is converted into families of interferons. These substances, in turn, have powerful antiviral actions.

Delta-6-desaturase

The last section might have left you slightly puzzled. How, you might be asking yourself, do viral infections ever manage to get a foothold in our bodies if they are susceptible to destruction by EPA? One key part of the answer is that in order to establish themselves in human bodies, viruses such as the Epstein Barr virus need to stop our bodies from producing eicosanoids, and, in particular, EPA.

Suppose you were the general in command of a viral invasion force. Where are the weakest parts of the human line of defence that you should try to hit? If you turn back to Figure 13, you will readily see that if a viral species were to block the very first enzyme that our cells use to manufacture long-chain polyunsaturated fatty acids, then it would effectively block the production of all eicosanoids and would, in particular, block the synthesis of EPA. This would mean that the human body would not be able to use its EPA-based defences against the invading viruses.

This is precisely what such viruses do. They stop that first enzyme (which you may remember is called delta-6-desaturase) from working properly, and so the cells and tissues of the human body are left essentially defenceless against the onslaught from the invading viruses, which are now free to reproduce rapidly and wreak havoc on the 'host'.

It is not just viruses that can block the action of the enzyme delta-6-desaturase. In the next section (Blocking the action of delta-6-desaturase, page 86) I shall describe other commonly occurring factors that can inhibit the action of this important enzyme. Whatever the cause of this inhibition, the result is that unless there is an intake of long-chain polyunsaturated fatty acids (principally GLA, AA and EPA) the body is deprived of these important fatty acids. In the year 2000, Dr Alex Richardson, from the University of Oxford, and I published a theoretical paper showing that some of the important features of ADHD can be accounted for by an underlying abnormality of fatty acid synthesis in which there are just such deficiencies. Let me explain.

The fatty acid model (Richardson and Puri)

As just mentioned, the fatty acid model of ADHD was put forward by Alex Richardson and me in a paper entitled 'The potential role of fatty acids in attention-deficit/hyperactivity disorder', published in the journal *Prostaglandins Leukotrienes and Essential Fatty Acids* in July/August 2000. Before going into further details of this model, let me start with a summary This is provided by the 'abstract' at the beginning of our paper:

As currently defined, attention-deficit/hyperactivity disorder (ADHD) encompasses a broad constellation of behavioural and learning problems and its definition and diagnosis remain controversial. The aetiology [cause] of ADHD is acknowledged to be both complex and multifactorial. The proposal considered here is that at least some features of ADHD may reflect an underlying abnormality of fatty acid metabolism. Clinical and biochemical evidence is discussed which suggests that a functional deficiency of certain long-chain polyunsaturated fatty acids could contribute to many of the features associated with this condition. The implications in terms of fatty acid treatment proposals are also discussed; such a form of treatment is relatively safe compared to existing pharmacological interventions, although further studies are still needed in order to evaluate its potential efficacy in the management of ADHD symptoms. (Reprinted from Richardson and Puri (2000), with permission from Elsevier.)

Blocking the action of delta-6-desaturase

In addition to viral infections, mentioned earlier, factors that can block the action of the enzyme delta-6-desaturase (see Figure 13) include:

- Saturated fats

- Hydrogenated fats including trans fats

- Deficiency of vitamin and mineral cofactors

- Excessive alcohol consumption, and

- Stress hormones.

Some of these factors, though I hope not the excessive consumption of alcohol, are common in children in the western world.

Their diets are often rich in saturated fats from meat products such as burgers and sausages. 'Foodstuffs' as diverse as bread and 'soft' ice cream may contain hydrogenated vegetable 'oils' that are rich in artificial manufactured trans fats. Certain vitamins and minerals act as important 'cofactors' in helping the fatty acids to be used by the body in the right way; some of these vitamins and minerals, such as zinc, may be deficient in modern diets.

Furthermore, the consumption of foods containing refined (white or coloured) sugar, refined (white or 'brown') flour, and white (polished) rice, also has a major detrimental effect. These refined 'foods' are depleted of vital vitamins and minerals. For example, in the manufacture of crystals of white sugar (chemically known as sucrose), all the vitamins, minerals and proteins are removed. In fact, around 90% of the sugar cane or sugar beet is taken away. However, for the body properly to digest the white sugar, white flour or white rice, some of these minerals and vitamins are needed. And so the body leaches these precious minerals and vitamins in order to try to cope with these artificially refined products. Needless to say, these refined products are abundant in the modern diet of most children in the western world, in products as diverse as sweets, sweetened fizzy drinks, cakes, biscuits, pastries and rice pudding. Even many manufactured foodproducts not immediately thought of as being sweet have white sugar hidden in them, such as baked beans and tomato ketchup.

Sadly, as children get older, they encounter increasing levels of stress, and with that, increasing levels of the stress hormone cortisol. This stress hormone circulates throughout the body and inhibits the action of delta-6-desaturase. I will say more about it in the final chapter.

(How can you counteract these factors? In later chapters I shall have more to say about trans fats (or trans fatty acids) and how they are manufactured. Meanwhile, the whole of Chapter 8 is devoted to a discussion of the cofactors, explaining which vitamins and minerals in particular help us to use fatty acids effectively and how to obtain them from our diet. If at all possible, you should try to wean your children off refined 'foods'. This means avoiding products containing white (refined) sugar, replacing white flour with wholemeal flour, and replacing white rice with whole grain unpolished 'brown' rice. The issue of stress hormones is dealt with in the final chapter.)

These potential blocks to conversion mean that a deficiency in GLA, AA and EPA can easily occur despite the essential fatty acid precursors (LA and ALA) being available in our diet. Without sufficient delta-6-desaturase we can make no use of them.

Let us now look at how this model is consistent with some of the key features of ADHD.

Abnormal brain functioning

The production of omega-3 and omega-6 fatty acids influences many aspects of brain development, including the migration of brain cells (the movement of brain cells during growth of the brain), the growth of nerve fibres, the branching of brain cells, and the creation, remodelling and pruning of connections between brain cells (Crawford, 1992). Animal studies have shown that the integrity and function of brain cells can be permanently disrupted by omega-3 and omega-6 fatty acid deficiencies during early development in the womb and just after birth (Yamamoto and colleagues, 1987; Neuringer and colleagues, 1988; Bourre and colleagues, 1989).

Blocking the action of the enzyme delta-6-desaturase means that cell membranes cannot get enough AA and DHA and consequently become more rigid, losing their normal flexibility. The effects on the protein receptor molecules that lie in the cell membranes (see Figure 10) are profound; the size and shape of these receptors change so that they no longer accept and pass on signals in the right way. This in turn damages communication between cells. The results of this in the human brain are 'cognitive defects', or problems with thought processes, such as short-term memory, attention and concentration, as seen in ADHD.

Genetics

Individuals differ in their in-built ability to convert the essential fatty acids LA and ALA into long-chain polyunsaturated fatty acids. This may mean there is a genetic component to the efficiency of this conversion process. Whether or not some of the same genes are involved in ADHD must remain speculative at this stage.

Neurotransmitters and neurotransmission

We saw in the last chapter that there is some evidence to suggest that abnormalities of dopamine neurotransmission may be involved in ADHD. I have already mentioned that the functioning of all neurotransmitters and their receptors can be strongly influenced by the lipid content of the membranes within which those receptors lie. Experiments have demonstrated that subtle changes to the fatty acids in phospholipid molecules in cell membranes (see Figures 10 and 11) can lead to profound changes in the ability of receptors to receive neurotransmitters. Furthermore, omega-3 and omega-6 long-chain polyunsaturated fatty acids are involved in many aspects of receptor function and of the synthesis and breakdown of neurotransmitters.

Still with me? The important message is that fatty acids are very important in the communication between our cells because of their relationship with neurotransmitters and their receptors. This communication of course includes the dopamine pathway that has been implicated in ADHD, as described in chapter 4. Do low levels of omega-3 fatty acids in fact lead to reduced activity of the neurotransmitter dopamine? There are several animal studies related to fatty acids, carried out in France, that are relevant.

A series of experiments on rats given diets deficient in omega-3 fatty acids has been carried out at the Laboratoire de Biophysique Médicale et Pharmaceutique in Tours, France, by the team of Dr Sylvie Chalon, in collaboration with Georges Durand of the Laboratoire de Nutrition et Sécurité Alimentaire in Jouy-en-Josas, France. These experiments have shown that a long-term deficiency of omega-3 fatty acids alters dopamine neurotransmission in the brain, with decreased levels of dopamine available at synapses in the frontal cortex. Further experiments by these teams, published in the *American Journal of Clinical Nutrition* by Zimmer and colleagues in 2002, have shown that omega-3 long-chain polyunsaturated fatty acid deficiency is related to changes in the dopamine pathways, with the result that the mesocortical system is less active. (This system was described in the previous chapter where it is shown diagrammatically in Figure 8.) So these findings show that the results of omega-3 deficiency, at least in the rat brain, tie in well with current thinking about the role of impaired dopamine neurotransmission in ADHD.

Thus, in the Richardson and Puri fatty acid model of ADHD, the fatty acid abnormalities are primary, while the neurotransmitter changes, including the abnormalities in dopamine neurotransmission, are secondary to this.

Gender

In Chapter 3 I mentioned that ADHD is more common in boys. You may recall that the most up-to-date figures for the male to female ratio in the community suggest that boys are about two-and-a-half times as likely as girls to suffer from ADHD. Our fatty acid model provides a ready explanation. Quoting our paper (Richardson and Puri, 2000) but omitting the references:

> While difficult to explain on the basis of a neurotransmitter model, this clinical observation is readily explicable by a fatty acid model, as males are more vulnerable than females to LC-PUFA deficiency. A similar excess of males is found in other developmental disorders that show clinical and familial associations with ADHD and with each other, including dyslexia, dyspraxia, and schizophrenia, and there is evidence implicating abnormalities of fatty acid metabolism in these disorders. (Reprinted from Richardson and Puri (2000) with permission from Elsevier.)

Minor physical abnormalities

ADHD is associated with an excess of minor physical abnormalities. These abnormalities include:

- Eyes that are more widely set than is usual

- Ears that have an unusual shape, and

- The creases on the palm of the hand (beloved of palm

readers or cheiromancers) show only one major palm crease rather than the usual two; that is the 'head' and 'heart' lines are more likely to be joined into one instead of being separate.

These findings are readily explicable by our fatty acid model. The spacing of the eyes, the shape of the ears and the creases of the palms involve the following processes:

- Cell remodelling (in which the structure of cells is changed)

- Programmed cell death (known as apoptosis), and

- Cell migration.

It turns out that phospholipid molecules, long-chain poly-unsaturated fatty acids and their derivatives have important parts to play in these processes. Abnormalities in fatty acids could therefore cause these minor physical abnormalities. Interestingly, there appears to be evidence that such abnormalities are also more common in certain other conditions (such as schizophrenia) that may be associated with fatty acid abnormalities.

Sleep problems

Children with ADHD are more likely than normal children to suffer from problems with sleep. These may include:

- Problems settling first thing at night

- Waking during the night, and

- Feeling over-tired in the morning.

The fatty acid model has a ready explanation for this. If the delta-6-desaturase enzyme is blocked, then insufficient levels of long-chain polyunsaturated fatty acids are synthesized by the body. Unable to make sufficient quantities of EPA, the human body is no longer able to manufacture sufficient quantities of the EPA-based natural sleep mediators. As a result, the body does not get enough deep refreshing sleep and ends up feeling tired.

Taking long-chain polyunsaturated fatty acids also makes cell membranes more fluid, as mentioned above. In turn, this means that ion channels and neurotransmitter receptors in brain cell membranes work better. Again, this leads to better and deeper sleep.

In 1989, a French team (Fagioli, Baroncini, Ricour and Salzarulo) from the INSERM in Paris published an interesting paper in the journal *Sleep*. They studied the sleep patterns of 15 children who were fed by 'total parenteral nutrition'. Total parenteral nutrition, also known as TPN, involves no feeding at all by mouth. Instead, the nutrients required are obtained by injection, usually through a 'drip' feed. In this study, the feeds of eight of the children did not include essential fatty acids, whereas those of the remaining seven children did include essential fatty acids. Fagioli and colleagues found that the level of an important constituent of normal sleep, known as slow-wave sleep, was noticeably reduced in the eight children who were not receiving dietary essential fatty acids, compared with the seven children who did receive their complement of essential fatty acids. This reduction was particularly noticeable during the second half of the night. Slow-wave sleep (which consists of 'stage 3' and 'stage 4' sleep) corresponds to deep sleep, and it is important that this deep sleep takes place if the person is to feel refreshed in the morning. This study illustrates the importance of lipids in obtaining deep, refreshing sleep.

Allergies and related health problems
Amongst the chronic health problems that have been found to be more common in children with ADHD than in normal children are:

- Upper respiratory tract (nose and throat) problems

- Allergies

- Skin disorders, and

- Asthma.

Some of these conditions, such as eczema, have now been shown often to be associated with a reduction in the efficiency with which the enzyme delta-6-desaturase works. In fact, this may be a problem with most allergic reactions. The result, of course, is that the body will have difficulty in converting linoleic acid and alpha-linolenic acid into important long-chain polyunsaturated fatty acids such as dihomo-gamma-linolenic acid (DGLA), AA and EPA. You will recall that these three long-chain polyunsaturated fatty acids in particular are the starting points for the synthesis, by the body, of the various families of important naturally occurring substances known collectively as eicosanoids. In turn, some of these eicosanoids play an extremely important part in the immune system and in (preventing) allergic reactions.

Other physical symptoms

Physical (or 'somatic') symptoms that are more common in children with ADHD than in normal children include:

- Headaches

- Stomach-aches

- Susceptibility to infections, and

- General malaise without an obvious cause.

Again, a lack of DGLA, AA and EPA would mean that the body cannot produce enough eicosanoids, and so the general health and well-being of the body would suffer. Without sufficient eicosanoids the body cannot mount proper immune response measures against infectious invading agents (such as bacteria and viruses), and may have to endure bouts of painful sore throats, and enlarged and tender neck (cervical) and armpit (axillary) lymph glands. Certain long-chain polyunsaturated fatty acids and their eicosanoid derivatives also play an important part in the regulation of digestive functions.

EPA and certain eicosanoids normally help to keep our joints working properly and 'well-oiled'. Their disappearance means that the body may have to endure pains (arthralgia) in many different joints. However, this does not usually manifest itself until adulthood.

Emotional and mood disorders

In Chapter 3 we saw how anxiety and depression may co-exist with ADHD, this phenomenon being known clinically as comorbidity. Indeed, studies that follow up what has happened to children with ADHD have established that the risk of depression during adolescence and young adulthood is increased. Interestingly, emotional and mood disorders may also occur more commonly than would otherwise be expected in the non-ADHD relatives of people with ADHD.

There is now ample evidence that a deficiency in omega-3 long-chain polyunsaturated fatty acids is associated with depression. This includes evidence from epidemiology, biochemistry, brain scans and clinical trials.

In 1998, Dr Joseph Hibbeln, a psychiatrist working in Maryland in the United States of America, published a paper in the *Lancet* in which he had looked at the annual rate of occurrence of clinical depression ('major depression') in nine countries. For those same nine countries, he had also examined the figures for the apparent annual fish consumption. These were estimated, for each country, by adding together the annual fish catch and annual imports of fish, and subtracting from this subtotal the annual fish exports. Surprisingly, the annual rate of depression was negatively correlated with the apparent fish consumption. That is, for countries with a low annual fish intake, such as New Zealand and West Germany (the data for the study came from before the fall of the Berlin Wall and the Soviet Union), the annual rate of occurrence of depression was high. Conversely, for countries with a high annual fish intake, such as Taiwan and Japan, the annual rate of occurrence of depression was low. Since oily fish are rich in omega-3 long-chain polyunsaturated fatty acids such as EPA, these results were consistent with an association between a lack of these fatty acids and the occurrence of depression. Since then, Joe Hibbeln and his colleagues have found a similar negative correlation between the annual seafood consumption for various countries, and both the lifetime rate of occurrence of bipolar mood disorder ('manic-depression') and of postnatal depression (depression occurring after childbirth).

In 1993, Professor Michael Maes and his colleagues published their analyses of the national Belgian data on suicide, violent suicide, non-violent suicide, and homicide for the period 1979 to 1987. They found a seasonal variation in depression and in violent suicide (that is, suicide by violent means, involving firearms, hanging, slashing or falls, as opposed, say, to drug overdoses). In 2004, the same group (De Vriese, Christophe and Maes) published a paper in the prestigious scientific journal *Prostaglandins Leukotrienes and Essential Fatty Acids* showing that the level of EPA appeared to predict the rate of violent suicide two weeks later; when the level of EPA was low, the rate of violent suicide was high a fortnight later, and *vice versa*.

On the biochemical front, a number of studies by different groups have shown that the level of EPA is low in the red blood cells of people who are depressed. Furthermore, some of these studies have also looked at the severity of depression, and found a negative correlation between the level of EPA and the severity of the depression; the lower the EPA level, the greater the severity of the depression, and *vice versa*. (The levels of EPA and other long-chain polyunsaturated fatty acids in red blood cells give a good indication of the corresponding levels in the brain. In theory, the incorporation (or, alternatively loss) of omega-3 and omega-6 fatty acids into the membranes of brain cells is reflected by a similar incorporation (or loss) into the membranes of all other living cells in the body. This includes the red blood cells, which, unlike brain cells, are readily accessible through the relatively simple and routine procedure of taking a blood sample.)

My group was the first to use brain scans to examine the effects of EPA treatment on the central nervous system. The results in depression have been extensively described in *The Natural Way to Beat Depression: The Groundbreaking Discovery of EPA to Change Your Life*, co-written with my colleague Hilary Boyd.

Using state-of-the-art brain imaging software applied to high-resolution brain scans, we found that not only did EPA noticeably improve severe depression, anxiety and social phobia, but it also actually caused the brain to re-grow (Puri and colleagues, 2001; 2002).

There have now been several large-scale clinical studies that have shown that EPA is an effective antidepressant. (EPA does not have the adverse side-effects associated with all the current classes of synthetic drug treatment for depression.) These trials have taken place in countries as diverse as England (Peet and Horrobin, 2002), Israel (Nehmets and colleagues, 2002) and Taiwan (Su and colleagues, 2003). In the first two of these studies, pure EPA was added to the current treatment of depressed patients who were not responding to their antidepressant therapy, while in the third study a mixture of EPA and DHA was used. In all three studies, there was a comparison group which received dummy (placebo) capsules, and in all three studies the group treated with omega-3 showed noticeable clinical improvement compared with the placebo group.

Learning disabilities

As I mentioned in Chapter 3, another set of disorders that often co-exist with ADHD are specific learning difficulties or language difficulties. These include dyslexia. As I said, this can make it even more difficult for children with ADHD to cope at school. Indeed, it is common for reading to be delayed in ADHD. The clinical over-lap between ADHD and dyslexia has been estimated to stand at 30% to 50% in both directions. That is, 30% to 50% of people with ADHD have dyslexia, and 30% to 50% of people with dyslexia have ADHD.

In 1997, the results of the first study of dyslexia using a specialized brain scanning technique known as 31-phosphorus neurospectroscopy (or 31-P magnetic resonance spectroscopy) were published by Dr Alex Richardson, from the University of Oxford, Dr Jane Cox, Janet Sargentoni and me (the last three being from Hammersmith Hospital, London). Our study showed clear and direct evidence that fatty acids are involved in dyslexia. In 2003,

Dr Richardson, Dr Eva Cyhlarova (also from Oxford University) and I published details of the clinical and biochemical fatty acid abnormalities in dyslexia. Fatty acids can also be used to help treat dyslexia (Richardson, 2003).

Biochemical evidence for fatty acid deficiency in ADHD

Blood studies

In our paper proposing the fatty acid hypothesis, Dr Alex Richardson and I also detailed some of the direct biochemical evidence for fatty acid deficiency in ADHD. I would now like to summarize this.

Mitchell and colleagues, working in North America, compared 48 hyperactive children with a 'control' group of 49 non-hyperactive children. The two groups were 'matched' (made as equal as possible) in terms of average age and gender. In their 1987 paper, published in the journal *Clinical Pediatrics*, the researchers found that significantly more of the hyperactive children (compared with the normal controls) suffered from:

- Auditory (hearing) difficulties

- Visual problems

- Language difficulties

- Reading difficulties

- Learning difficulties

- Frequent coughs and colds

- Thirst

- Passing urine more frequently, and

- A serious illness or accident in the previous year.

Feeling thirsty and passing urine more often can be caused by fatty acid deficiency. The researchers also found that the birth weight of the hyperactive children, at an average of 3.058 kg, was lower than that of the normal comparison group (average birth weight 3.410 kg). The researchers measured the blood levels of fatty acids in 44 of the hyperactive children and in 45 of the normal control children. They found that the average levels of certain omega-3 and omega-6 fatty acids were significantly lower in the hyperactive children. In particular, the average levels of the omega-6 long-chain polyunsaturated fatty acids DGLA (dihomo-gamma-linolenic acid) and AA (arachidonic acid) were lower, as was the average level of the omega-6 fatty acid DHA (docosahexaenoic acid).

The team of Laura Stevens and John Burgess, from the Department of Foods and Nutrition of Purdue University in Indiana, in the United States, published a similar study in 1995. In their research paper in the *American Journal of Clinical Nutrition*, they described how they had compared the plasma and red blood cell levels of omega-3 and omega-6 fatty acids in 53 boys with ADHD with the corresponding levels in 43 normal non-ADHD boys (who constituted the control group). The two groups were matched for average age. Compared with the control group, on average the 53 boys with ADHD:

- were less likely to have been breastfed (breast milk contains preformed long-chain polyunsaturated fatty acids, while most formula preparations do not)

- were more likely to suffer from allergies and other health problems (which, as mentioned above, are known to be associated with fatty acid deficiency)

- showed clinical signs of fatty acid deficiency (such as increased thirst, passing urine more frequently, dry skin and dry hair)

- showed reduced blood levels of certain long-chain polyunsaturated fatty acids (in plasma: reduced AA, EPA, DHA and total omega-3 fatty acids; and in red blood cell membranes: reduced AA and adrenic acid but increased omega-6 docosapentaenoic acid, which typically accumulates when there is a deficiency of omega-3 fatty acids)

- showed no deficiency in the essential fatty acid precursors of these omega-3 and omega-6 long-chain polyunsaturated fatty acids (that is, there was no deficiency in LA or ALA), and

- had an adequate dietary intake of the essential fatty acid precursors (LA and ALA).

These results suggest that at least some of these children with ADHD had difficulty in converting the essential fatty acid precursors (LA and ALA) into long-chain polyunsaturated fatty acids such as AA and EPA (see Figure 13). Overall, around 40% of the children with ADHD had a greater frequency of symptoms and signs consistent with fatty acid deficiency compared with just 9% of the non-ADHD children. The symptoms and signs of fatty acid deficiency found by these same researchers were:

- Increased thirst

- Frequent urination

- High fluid consumption, and

- Dry hair.

These symptoms and signs also apply to adults who are fatty acid deficient. From my clinical experience, other features of deficiency include:

- Dry skin

- 'Follicular keratoses' – a group of skin diseases in which the skin can be rough and hard, and/or itchy, sometimes with fissuring and discolouration

- Dry lips

- Dandruff

- Problematic nails – either brittle or too soft

- Sleep problems

- Frequent coughs and colds

- Allergies, asthma, and the like

- Excessively cold hands when the external temperature is not found to be too cold by others, and

- Excessively cold feet when the external temperature is not found to be too cold by others.

A further interesting study by Laura Stevens' group was published in the journal *Physiology and Behavior* in 1996. The aim of this study was to compare behaviour, learning and health problems in boys aged 6 to 12 years who had low plasma levels of total omega-3 and omega-6 fatty acids with boys in the same age range who had higher levels of these fatty acids. The researchers found that, on average, the boys with the low plasma omega-3 and omega-6 fatty acids had:

- A higher frequency of symptoms indicating fatty acid deficiency (as reported by their parents)

- A greater number of behavioural problems (as assessed using a specialized rating scale known as the Conners' Rating Scale, which we shall meet again in the next section of this chapter)

- Increased temper tantrums

- Increased levels of sleep problems – particularly marked in those with low omega-3 fatty acid levels, who had greater problems in getting off to sleep and greater problems getting up in the morning

- More learning problems, and

- Increased health problems, including suffering more colds and having a history of using more antibiotics.

Teachers were asked to evaluate the academic skills of the children. They found that those children with specifically low omega-3 fatty acid levels scored significantly lower on mathematics and overall academic ability compared with those boys who had high omega-3 fatty acid levels. Boys with low omega-3 fatty acid levels also complained more of stomach-aches than did boys with high omega-3 levels.

A further study, this time in Turkey, was carried out by Bekaroglu and colleagues and published in the *Journal of Child Psychology and Psychiatry* in 1996. This group, from the Department of Psychiatry at Technical University in Trabzon, Turkey, reported that, compared with 45 healthy children matched for age and gender, the average level of fatty acids in the blood serum (the liquid part of blood in which the red and white cells are carried) of 48 children with ADHD was significantly lower. They also found that the average level of zinc in the serum of the children with ADHD (just under 61 micrograms per decilitre) was also significantly lower than that in the control group of non-ADHD children (at just under 106 micrograms per decilitre). In fact, they found that there was a positive correlation between the level of zinc and the fatty acid levels in the ADHD children. In other words, the lower the zinc level, the lower the fatty acid level. You will recall how earlier in this book we saw that a lack of zinc can inhibit the functioning of the enzyme delta-6-desaturase and so prevent the body from making omega-3 and omega-6 long-chain polyunsaturated fatty acids (such as DGLA, AA and EPA).

A study by Jiun-Rong Chen and colleagues published in 2004 looked at ADHD in children in Taiwan. It was carried out by the Department of Nutrition and Health Sciences of Taipei Medical University, in collaboration with Taiwan Adventist Hospital and the Yuanpei Institute of Science and Technology. The researchers studied 58 children with ADHD and compared them with 52 normal non-ADHD children matched for age and gender (the control group). Compared with the control group, the average levels of AA and DHA in red blood cell membranes were significantly lower in the children with ADHD. The total levels of omega-3 fatty acids in red blood cell membranes were also lower in the children with ADHD. The diets of the children were also studied, and no significant difference was found between the groups in their intake of the essential fatty acid precursors of omega-3 and omega-6 acids (ALA and LA, respectively). Again, these results point to a possible problem in ADHD with the conversion of essential (short-chain) fatty acids into the long-chain polyunsaturated fatty acids.

The first study of blood fatty acids in adults with ADHD was published in 2004, in the journal *Lipids*, by a group based at the Department of Human Biology and Nutritional Sciences of the University of Guelph in Ontario, Canada. Young, Maharaj and Conquer studied 37 adults with ADHD and compared them with 35 non-ADHD adults. The adults with ADHD had significantly lower levels of DHA and of total omega-6 fatty acids in their blood serum (the liquid part of blood). In their red blood cell membranes, the adults with ADHD had significantly lower levels of total omega-3 fatty acids (including DHA) compared with the non-ADHD control group. So the fatty acid results noted in childhood ADHD also seem to apply to adult ADHD.

Breath study

We have seen clear evidence that omega-3 and omega-6 long-chain polyunsaturated fatty acids are deficient in both childhood ADHD and adult ADHD. Since the corresponding essential fatty acid precursors (ALA and LA) are not deficient in ADHD, and since there is evidence of a deficiency in zinc (which is needed for the proper functioning of delta-6-desaturase), it seems likely that a major cause of the deficiency of omega-3 and omega-6 long-chain polyunsaturated fatty acids is a block in the ability of the body to produce them from ALA and LA. In other words, it is likely that the enzyme delta-6-desaturase is being inhibited in some way.

There is another factor that might also be playing a part in these omega-3 and omega-6 fatty acid deficiencies. It could be that these long-chain polyunsaturated fatty acids (including EPA and DGLA) are being broken down to a greater extent in ADHD. This possibility can now be investigated using a safe, non-invasive technique, which involves simply collecting a sample of a person's breath.

When certain long-chain polyunsaturated fatty acids break down, as a result, say, of 'oxidative stress' they give rise to 'breakdown products'. Oxidative stress is observed in everyday life. For instance, when an apple is halved and left in the air, the area exposed to the oxygen in the atmosphere turns brown. A chemical in the apple has been 'oxidised'. Again, butter left in the open air at room temperature will become rancid. Oxidative stress causes destruction of lipid molecules because too much oxygen can be dangerous; the oxygen molecules can readily turn into free radicals. These may be involved in various degenerative and ageing processes; the body tries to protect itself from these oxidant effects by using antioxidants such as vitamin C.

The body eliminates some of the breakdown products from oxidative damage to brain fatty acids in your breath. The levels in breath are exceedingly small, but these days they can be detected accurately, using state-of-the-art techniques. The collected breath is passed through a machine known as a gas chromatograph mass spectrometer (or GCMS for short). This gives rise to a breath chemical 'fingerprint' that gives accurate information regarding different compounds in the breath. Using appropriate software, it is also possible to determine the amounts of some of those compounds that are present.

The first application of such technology to ADHD was by the Ness Foundation, part of the University of the Highlands and Islands Millennium Institute, based in Inverness, Scotland. The levels of ethane were measured in the exhaled (breathed out) breath of 10 children with ADHD and in 12 volunteers. Ethane is a particular breakdown product from oxidative damage to omega-3 fatty acids and therefore a useful indicator of the level of that oxidative damage within an individual. The group of researchers (Ross, McKenzie, Glen and Bennett) found that the average ethane level was higher in the ADHD group (indicating a greater level of oxidative damage to omega-3 fatty acids) than in the normal control group. In contrast, the groups showed no significant difference in the average levels of a different chemical that results from the oxidation of protein, indicating that the differences in oxidative damage were not general but specific to omega-3 fatty acids. In other words, this study, published in 2003 in *Nutritional Neuroscience*, suggests that in ADHD there may be specific oxidative break down of omega-3 long-chain polyunsaturated fatty acids.

If we now bring this evidence for greater break down of omega-3 fatty acids together with the evidence for patients with ADHD having difficulty in synthesizing long-chain polyunsaturated fatty acids in the first place from their essential fatty acid precursors we can draw an important conclusion. If patients with ADHD are deficient in omega-3 and omega-6 fatty acids because they can't synthesize enough and what they can synthesize is broken down too quickly to be useful, the appropriate treatment to try for ADHD would be supplements containing the deficient long-chain polyunsaturated fatty acids.

I shall now look at the clinical studies that have been carried out so far, which have attempted to treat ADHD with long-chain polyunsaturated fatty acids.

Fatty acid treatment studies

Several studies, or 'trials', of long-chain polyunsaturated fatty acids have now taken place. I have divided them up into the early ones that used evening primrose oil alone, one that used DHA alone, one that used predominantly DHA without omega-6 long-chain polyunsaturated fatty acids, and recent ones using a mixture of omega-3 long-chain polyunsaturated fatty acids including EPA and evening primrose oil (or equivalent). You do not need to remember all the details, as at the end of this chapter I will summarize the findings. Then in Chapter 6, I will give a brief, practical guide to taking fatty acid supplements for ADHD.

Before we look at the results of the studies, or trials, themselves, we need to look at the meaning of two terms: double-blind trials; and statistical significance. If you find mathematics a little daunting, then please feel free to omit the subsection on statistical significance; you should still be able to understand the material that follows it.

Double-blind trials

In a 'double-blind placebo-controlled trial', patients are allocated at random into two or more groups. The random allocation can be done on the basis of tossing a coin, or by using a table of random numbers, or by using a computer random number generator, for example. Those who are allocated to receive the putative treatment (the fatty acids, in this case) are said to be in an 'active' group. The 'active' treatment is compared with a dummy treatment, known as the placebo. This is to take into account the placebo effect, the improvement in symptoms that can arise simply because the patient thinks he or she is receiving a treatment. The placebo treatment consists of capsules (or tablets, etc) that are identical in appearance to the active treatment. Including the placebo group makes the trial 'placebo-controlled'.

In a double-blind study, neither the patients nor the clinicians or other researchers assessing them are aware of the group allocation (active or placebo) until the end of the trial, hence the term 'double-blind'.

The gold standard for research in pharmacology these days is the randomized double-blind placebo-controlled trial.

Statistical significance

I have used the terms 'significant' and 'significantly' in this chapter in relation to the results of blood studies and the breath study of ADHD. In addition to their usual English-language meanings, these words also convey 'statistical significance'. I shall now explain what this means.

When scientists say that a finding is statistically significant, they mean that the result found was unlikely to have occurred by chance. Let us look at a rather contrived example. Normally if you toss an unbiased or fair coin in the air, then all things being equal there is a one in two chance that it will land with the head uppermost ('heads'). There is also a corresponding one in two chance that it will land as 'tails'. (For purposes of simplicity, I am here ignoring the slight chance that the coin might land on its edge.) Now suppose you are given a biased coin that is weighted to make it come up 'heads'. You are asked to check whether or not this coin is biased. Suppose, further, that the only way you are allowed to carry out this test is by tossing the coin. Well, you toss the coin once, and the result is heads. This does not really prove anything at all, as there is a one in two chance that you would have got heads if the coin were unbiased. However, if you toss the coin three times, you will get a result of three consecutive heads. A question you could now ask yourself is: 'How likely is it that I could get three or more consecutive heads purely by chance if the coin is unbiased?' Well, the chances of getting one head purely by chance with a fair coin are one in two, or one-half. So the chances of getting three heads purely by chance with a fair coin are (one-half) times (one-half) times (one-half). This is one-eighth. So there is a one in eight chance of getting a result of three consecutive heads (or a more extreme result – that is, more than three consecutive heads) purely by chance if the coin is unbiased. Most scientists would consider that a chance of one in eight is well within the bounds of everyday possibility. The threshold that scientists set for considering that a result is unlikely to have occurred purely by chance tends to be around one in 20. (For those familiar with scientific papers, this is the origin of the famous 'P is less than 0.05' statement of statistical significance. The P stands for the probability (or chances) of the result occurring by chance. The 0.05 is the decimal representation of the fraction 1/20, which is the same as 'one in 20'.)

Suppose now that you decide to carry out a much better trial to test whether or not the coin is fair by tossing it 10 times. This time, the biased coin lands heads uppermost on ten consecutive occasions. The likelihood that this might happen by chance is:

(1/2) times (1/2) times (1/2) times (1/2) times (1/2) times (1/2) times (1/2) times (1/2) times (1/2) times (1/2).

This equals 1/1024. In other words, this result (or a more extreme result) has a less than one in a thousand likelihood of occurring by chance. Now you really would have reason to suspect that the coin might be biased. Of course, the more times you toss the coin, the more accurate your assessment will be; but in practice there is a limit to how far you can go. In a similar fashion, in scientific studies, there are practical factors that limit how far you can proceed. For example, in the studies of blood from people with ADHD that I have just described, the researchers would have got more accurate results if they had taken blood samples from every single person with ADHD in the whole world during a one-week period. This was clearly not practical. Similarly, when checking whether or not a coin is biased, you would obtain a higher accuracy if you were to spend your whole life tossing the coin every second of every day.

Evening primrose oil alone

You will recall that gamma-linolenic acid (GLA) is an omega-6 long-chain polyunsaturated fatty acid that is derived from linoleic acid (LA) through the action of the enzyme delta-6-desaturase (see Figure 13). Our bodies require dihomo-gamma-linolenic acid (DGLA) and arachidonic acid (AA), and as you can see from Figure 13, GLA can be converted into DGLA, which in turn can be converted into AA. (Neither of these last two reactions requires delta-6-desaturase.) So, if the action of delta-6-desaturase is inhibited, we can provide the fatty acids required by by-passing the linoleic acid stage and taking GLA.

At the time of writing, there have been two randomized double-blind placebo-controlled trials to see if ADHD/hyperactivity can be treated with GLA. In each case, the source of GLA has been evening primrose oil.

Aman, Mitchell and Turbott's study

The first randomized double-blind placebo-controlled trial of GLA was published in the *Journal of Abnormal Child Psychology* by Aman, Mitchell and Turbott in 1987. In this study, 31 children suffering from inattention and hyperactivity were randomly allocated to receive either evening primrose oil or a placebo for four weeks.

As might be expected from what I have discussed already, patients taking the evening primrose oil supplement saw an increase in their levels of DGLA. They also did two tasks significantly better based on parent ratings of attention problems and of excess motor activity. However, these same patients showed no significant improvements in eight other psychomotor (psychological and motor) performance tasks, nor in two standardized teacher rating scales.

Overall, although the authors concluded that taking evening primrose oil as a supplement produced minimal or no improvements in hyperactive children, it should be noted that the hyperactive children took evening primrose oil for only four weeks, and without the synergistic (supportive) potential benefits of the omega-3 fatty acid EPA. As Alex Richardson and I commented in the paper that set out our fatty acid model:

> Evidence gathered since then suggests that n-3 [omega-3] rather than n-6 [omega-6] fatty acid deficiency may be of more relevance in ADHD. Another fundamental issue is that the study design and treatment duration...cannot be considered appropriate for the evaluation of fatty acid treatment...[F]atty acids cannot be expected to act rapidly to change symptoms or behaviour. Rather, recent evidence has shown that LC-PUFA [long-chain polyunsaturated fatty acid] levels in the brain may take up to 3 months to recover from a chronic deficiency state, and this must therefore be regarded as an essential consideration in the design of future treatment studies. (Reprinted from Richardson and Puri (2000) with permission from Elsevier.)

The Ohio State University study

The second randomized double-blind placebo-controlled trial of evening primrose oil was carried out by the team of Arnold and colleagues from the Ohio State University in Columbus, USA.

It was published in 1989 in the journal *Biological Psychiatry* and involved a comparison of GLA (from evening primrose oil) against a placebo and also against *d*-amphetamine. Eighteen boys suffering from ADHD and aged between six and 12 years took part in the study. Using a particular variant of the double-blind trial called a Latin-square double-crossover study, each child received (in random sequence) one month of each of these three possible 'treatments' – namely, evening primrose oil, placebo, and *d*-amphetamine. Ratings of the boys with ADHD were collected from the teachers.

Taking evening primrose oil gave benefits on the teachers' ratings that were intermediate between those of *d*-amphetamine and the placebo. In the case of one of the factors studied, the Conners' Hyperactivity Factor, the differences were statistically significant (P less than 0.05). We shall describe the Conners' factors in more detail later in this chapter.

The authors concluded that this study did not establish evening primrose oil as an effective treatment. Again, the same weaknesses apply in this study as for the study by Aman and colleagues: there was no EPA used; and a one-month treatment regimen is too short for a clear therapeutic effect from fatty acids.

DHA alone

At the time of writing there has been one randomized double-blind placebo-controlled trial published which involved studying the effects of using DHA (the omega-6 long-chain polyunsaturated fatty acid docosahexaenoic acid) alone versus a placebo. This was the American study by Robert Voigt and colleagues, and involved a collaboration between the Division of Developmental and Behavioral Pediatrics of the Mayo Clinic in Rochester, Minnesota, and the Departments of Pediatrics, Psychiatry and the United States Department of Agriculture, Agricultural Research Service Children's Nutrition Research Center of the Baylor College of Medicine in Houston, Texas. The study was published in 2001 in the *Journal of Pediatrics*. Sixty-three children with ADHD aged between six and 12 years were randomly allocated to take part in this study. All were already receiving maintenance medication with stimulant therapy. The design of the study was such that for four months, the children additionally received either 345 milligrams daily of DHA (the active group) or else a placebo (the placebo group).

There tend to be 'drop-outs' in any large clinical study; patients may leave a study for all manner of reasons. This study was no exception. After discarding the results from those children who did not complete the full trial, there were 54 children who had completed the full four-months, 27 in the active (DHA) group and 27 in the placebo group. The two groups were statistically matched in terms of age, gender and ethnicity (that is, there was no significant difference between the groups in relation to these factors). They were also matched in terms of the maintenance treatment with psychostimulants being received. Of the 27 children in the DHA group, 25 were taking methylphenidate, one dextroamphetamine and one amphetamine/dextroamphetamine. The corresponding figures in the placebo group were 22, two and three. The average doses of these stimulant drugs did not differ significantly between the groups either.

The results and conclusion of the study were summarized as follows by Robert Voigt and colleagues:

Results: Plasma phospholipid DHA content of the DHA-supplemented group was 2.6-fold higher at the end of the study than that of the placebo group (4.85 ± 1.35 vs 0.87 mol % of total fatty acids; $P < 0.001$). Despite this, there was no statistically significant improvement in any objective or subjective measure of ADHD symptoms.

Conclusion: A 4-month period of DHA supplementation (345 milligrams/d) does not decrease symptoms of ADHD. (Reprinted from Voigt *et al* (2001) with permission from Elsevier.)

In fact, looking closely at the results, it appears that the DHA group actually fared worse than the placebo group (although the differences did not reach statistical significance) on parental measures of:

- Internalizing behaviours

- Externalizing behaviours

- Socialization problems

- Thought problems, and

- Attention problems.

On one set of psychological tests of attention and impulsivity, errors of commission were measured at baseline and four-month follow-up (at the end of the study). Whereas the DHA group showed no statistically significant difference between scores over four months, the placebo group actually showed more than a halving of errors on the test, a result that was highly statistically significant (P less than 0.0003).

Overall, then, this study indicates that it is definitely not a good idea to try to treat ADHD with DHA alone. There are, in fact, deeper reasons why DHA should be avoided in supplements. Not only is DHA not effective (and actually worse than a placebo on some measures, as seen in Robert Voigt's study), but, as we shall see in Chapter 6, there is accumulating evidence that supplements containing too much DHA may actually be harmful to health. Interestingly, these potential concerns are echoed by the following sentence in the paper by Voigt and colleagues:

> Indeed, despite a lack of data to support either efficacy or safety, DHA supplements are readily available and are being marketed for the treatment of children with ADHD. (Reprinted from Voigt *et al* (2001) with permission from Elsevier.)

High DHA, low EPA, no evening primrose oil

In 2004, a Japanese study was published under the title 'Effect of docosahexaenoic acid-containing [DHA-containing] food administration on symptoms of attention-deficit/hyperactivity disorder – a placebo-controlled double-blind study'. The authors of this trial, published in the *European Journal of Clinical Nutrition*, were Hirayama, Hamazaki and Terasawa. The study involved a collaboration between the Department of Early Childhood Education and Care at Kurashiki City College in Okayama and Toyama Medical and Pharmaceutical University in Toyama. It took place in a summer camp for children with psychiatric disorders run by Dr Hirayama.

The study involved 40 children with ADHD aged between six and 12 years who were randomly allocated to two groups. The study lasted two months. The active group, containing 20 of the children, had their diets supplemented by foods that had been enriched with fish oil. These consisted of a selection from fermented soybean milk, bread rolls and steamed bread. These fortified foods provided 514 milligrams DHA daily (3.6 grams of DHA per week). Since these foods had fish oil added to them, and since fish oil also contains EPA, there was also a small amount of EPA present too, namely 100 milligrams daily (700 milligrams of EPA per week). The placebo (control) group also consisted of 20 children, who received the same extra foods over two months, this time fortified with olive oil, which, unlike fish oil, does not contain DHA. Just two of the DHA group and four of the control group took stimulant medication during the course of the two-month study; all the other 34 children were medication-free. The two groups were matched for gender (16 boys and four girls in each group) and average age (nine years in each group).

Tests of short-term memory were carried out at the start and end of the study. Auditory short-term memory was tested by asking the children to listen to seven-digit numbers and then assessing how well they had remembered them straight afterwards. On average, the change in auditory short-term memory for the DHA group over the two months was actually worse than for the control group. (A statistical test of the difference between the DHA group and the control group on this test gave $P = 0.07$.) With the test of visual short-term memory, in which the children's memorizing ability after looking at seven-digit numbers for 10 seconds was assessed, the DHA group again fared worse than the control group over the two-month period. This time, while the control group improved by an average (actually the 'median') of one-and-a-half digits (from an average of three-and-a-half digits remembered correctly at the start of the study improving to an average of five digits correctly remembered at the end of the two months), the DHA group only improved by an average of half a digit (from an average of two-and-a-half digits remembered correctly at the start of the study rising only to an average of three digits correctly remembered at the end of the two months). The poor performance of the DHA group on the visual short-term memory test was even worse, statistically, than for the auditory short-term memory test, with the P value for the difference between the DHA group and the control group being 0.02.

If the negative action of DHA on visual and auditory short-term memory was not bad enough, the DHA group also fared worse than the control group on the children's ability to carry out a continuous performance test. In this test, one of the nine digits from one to nine was displayed on a computer screen for four seconds and then replaced by another digit. The children were asked to press a button only when they saw the sequence of number nine after number one (that is, only after seeing '...19'). Errors of omission (not pressing the button when this sequence occurred) and errors of commission (pressing the button when this sequence had not occurred) were measured. For the control group, the average ('median') number of errors of omission improved significantly ($P = 0.02$) over the two-month study period. In contrast, for the DHA group the number of errors of omission actually worsened over the same time interval. Similarly, for the control group, the average ('median') number of errors of commission improved significantly ($P = 0.01$) over the two-month period. Again, for the DHA group the number of errors of commission actually worsened over the same time period. (For the statistically minded, the difference between the improvement in the number of errors of commission for the control group and the deterioration for the DHA group was so great that the P value for the contrast between the two groups was just 0.001.)

On a standardized test of attention, the DHA group did show an improvement over the two-month period from an average (median) of four correct answers at baseline to ten by the end of the study. However, again the control group showed an even greater improvement over the same time period, from an average (median) of four-and-a-half to 15.

The researchers also rated the average number of symptoms according to DSM-IV (see Box 1 in Chapter 2; the symptoms in DSM-IV are the same as for DSM-IV-TR). Over the two-month period of the study, the average number of symptoms of attention deficit remained the same for the control group but actually increased for the DHA group (that is, the DHA group became worse, on average). Moreover, whereas the average number of symptoms of impulsivity remained the same over the two months for the DHA group, they actually fell for the control group (that is, again the control group fared better).

The authors were surprised by their results – DHA was worse than placebo. They wondered in their paper about several possible reasons for this. One was that perhaps olive oil was not the best choice of placebo. They quoted a letter that Dr Alex Richardson and I had published in the *Archives of General Psychiatry* (Puri and Richardson, 2000) to explain why olive oil might affect someone's mood. They went on to counter this argument by noting that less than 9 grams of olive oil per week had been used in the control foods, and that the main psychoactive fatty acid in olive oil, namely oleic acid, was already present in relatively large amounts in the body fat. In other words, they thought that the effects of the placebo oil were likely to be negligible.

Even more interesting was their considered suggestion that it would be worth trying pure EPA instead of DHA. They openly wondered what the effects on children with ADHD would be of using pure EPA rather than either DHA-containing fish oil or pure DHA. This was reinforced in their overall conclusion that DHA supplementation did not lead to improvement in any ADHD symptoms. In future studies, they argued, the particular fatty acids used should be chosen with care.

EPA, DHA and GLA (from evening primrose oil or equivalent)

The Purdue University study

The Purdue University study was a study by the group mentioned earlier that had investigated the levels of fatty acids in blood in ADHD children. In this four-month trial, published in 2003 in the journal *Lipids*, Laura Stevens, John Burgess and colleagues randomly allocated 50 children with ADHD-like symptoms to receive either a long-chain polyunsaturated fatty acid supplement or an olive oil placebo daily. The active group received the following daily doses:

- 480 milligrams DHA

- 80 milligrams EPA

- 96 milligrams GLA

- 40 milligrams AA.

In view of what we have just said about the negative actions of DHA, it was a shame that the active group received such a high dose of DHA. Just the following two out of 16 outcome measures showed any significant benefit for the active group:

- Conduct problems, rated by parents ($P = 0.05$)

- Attention symptoms, rated by teachers ($P = 0.03$).

Harding, Judah and Gant

This United States study was carried out by Dr Karen Harding (Harvard Medical School), Dr Richard Judah (Vermont College of Union Institute and University) and Dr Charles Gant (National Integrated Health Associates, Washington DC). Their paper, 'Outcome-based comparison of Ritalin® versus food-supplement treated children with AD/HD' was published in 2003 in the journal *Alternative Medicine Review*.

Twenty children with ADHD aged between seven and 12 years were divided into groups. Ten children made up the first group, and all of them received methylphenidate (in the form Ritalin®) for the whole four-week duration of the study, having not been taking it before the study began. The dose of this stimulant used varied between 5 and 15 milligrams two to three times daily. The other group received a large number of daily nutritional supplements that are listed in the box below. For the results of the study turn to page 120.

Box 5. Daily nutritional supplements taken by 10 children in the study by Harding, Judah and Gant

- For gastrointestinal and immune support

  Lactobacillus acidophilus

  Lactobacillus bifidus

  Silymarin 5 milligrams

- Sulphur (sulfur)–containing supplements and glycine

  Taurine 275 to 425 milligrams

  Glycine 700 to 1830 milligrams

  Methionine 25 to 75 milligrams

  N-acetylcysteine up to 10 milligrams

  L-cysteine up to 25 milligrams

  Glutathione 20 milligrams

  alpha Lipoic acid 5 milligrams

  Garlic extract 200 milligrams

- Other amino acids

  Tyrosine 900 to 1800 milligrams

  Histidine 25 to 75 milligrams

  Glutamine 600 to 1400 milligrams

  alpha Ketoglutarate 25 to 75 milligrams

  L-carnitine 30 milligrams

(Box 5 continued)

- Minerals

    Magnesium (as glycinate) 220 to 480 milligrams

    Calcium (as ascorbate) 110 to 170 milligrams

    Potassium (as glycerol phosphate) 46 to 70 milligrams

    Chromium (as nicotinate) 140 to 200 micrograms

    Selenium (as methionate) 26 to 32 micrograms

    Zinc (as monomethionate) 9 to 15 milligrams

    Manganese (as arginate) 2.5 to 4 milligrams

    Boron (as citrate) 1200 to 1800 micrograms

    Copper (as tyrosinate) 1.2 to 2.4 milligrams

    Silica 4 milligrams

    Molybdenum (as chelate) 5 to 40 micrograms

    Vanadium (as chelate) 2 to 20 micrograms

    Iron (as glycinate) 1 to 2 milligrams

- Fatty acids and phospholipids

    Salmon oil 1000 milligrams, providing 180 milligrams EPA and 120 milligrams DHA

    Borage oil 200 milligrams, providing 45 milligrams GLA

    Purified soy lecithin, providing 50 to 150 milligrams phosphatidyl choline and 20 to 25 milligrams inositol

    Choline bitartrate 2.5 to 7.5 milligrams

- Agents to support thyroid functioning

    Iodine (from kelp) 25 to 150 micrograms

    Tyrosine 900 to 1800 milligrams

- Vitamins and phytonutrients

    Vitamin B_1 (as thiamine and thiamine

(Box 5 continued)

pyrophosphate) 22.5 to 27.5 milligrams

Vitamin B_2 (as riboflavin and riboflavin phosphate) 22.5 to 27.5 milligrams

Vitamin B_3 (as niacin and niacinamide) 75 to 140 milligrams

Vitamin B_5 (as D-calcium pantothenate and pantethine) 50 to 70 milligrams

Vitamin B_6 (as pyridoxine and pyridoxal-5-phosphate) 43 to 86 milligrams

Vitamin B_{12} (cyanocobalamin) 90 to 175 micrograms

Folic acid 435 to 760 micrograms

Biotin 20 to 400 micrograms

PABA 22.5 to 27.5 milligrams

Vitamin E 140 to 200 IU

Vitamin C 750 to 1000 milligrams

Vitamin A (as vitamin A and beta carotene) 2000 to 4500 IU

Vitamin D_3 40 to 100 IU

Vitamin K 20 micrograms

Royal bee jelly (source of biopterin) 75 to 150 milligrams

Dimethyl glycine 10 milligrams

Citrus bioflavonoids 10 to 20 milligrams

Proanthocyanidins (grape seed) 5 milligrams

Bilberry extract 20 milligrams

Soy constituents (saponins, isoflavones, phytosterols) 20 milligrams

Overall, the results of this study suggested that the supplement used might be equal in efficacy to methylphenidate. In particular, the children in both the supplement group and those in the methylphenidate group showed significant improvement on several psychological measures of auditory (listening) and visual attention, and auditory and visual response.

Of the wide variety of supplements used in this study, the fatty acids were likely to have been of particular importance, as indicated by the next study.

Richardson and Puri

In 2002, Dr Alex Richardson, from the University of Oxford, and I published a paper with the title 'A randomized double-blind, placebo-controlled study of the effects of supplementation with highly unsaturated fatty acids on ADHD-related symptoms in children with specific learning difficulties', in the journal *Progress in Neuropsychopharmacology and Biological Psychiatry*. Forty-one children aged between eight and 12 years were recruited into this study. They were suffering from learning difficulties (mainly dyslexia) and also had ADHD symptoms. (You may recall from earlier in this book that ADHD and dyslexia show strong overlap, or comorbidity.) These children had been referred to a special school in Northern Ireland for children with specific literacy problems. None of the children took any stimulant medication during the study.

Twenty-two of the children were randomly allocated to the fatty acid treatment group, while the remaining 19 children were allocated to the placebo group. By the end of the 12-week study ratings were obtained for 29 of the children (15 active, 14 placebo); these two groups did not differ significantly with respect to age or sex. The active treatment consisted of the following daily fatty acid doses:

- EPA 186 milligrams

- DHA 480 milligrams

- GLA 96 milligrams

- LA 864 milligrams

- AA 42 milligrams.

The placebo used was olive oil. It was a pity that the active treatment contained so much DHA, but at the time of the study the preparation used was the one that contained the highest ratio of EPA to DHA, together with GLA, that was readily available to us.

Dr C Keith Conners developed some of the most widely used ADHD 'rating scales'. (A rating scale is a tool or instrument that is used to capture information about, in this case, the types and severity of ADHD symptoms and signs.) One of these, which was used in our study, is the Conners' Parent Rating Scale (CPRS-L) (Conners, 1997) in which parents are asked detailed questions about the severity of the different features of the ADHD that their child suffers from. At both baseline (before treatment started) and after 12 weeks the Conners' Parent Rating Scale was used to assess a range of behavioural and learning problems associated with ADHD. This yielded scores, standardized for age, for seven sub-scales assessing individual features of ADHD (Oppositional, Cognitive Problems, Hyperactivity, Anxious-Shy, Perfectionism, Social Problems, Psychosomatic) and seven global scales (Conners' ADHD Index, Conners' Restless-Impulsive, Conners' Emotional Lability, Conners' Global Total, DSM Inattention, DSM Hyperactive-Impulsive, DSM Global Total). Teacher rating scales of ADHD symptoms were not considered appropriate, since all the children were new to their school.

At the start of the study, the two groups did not differ significantly on any of the 14 scales. However, after 12 weeks the average scores for cognitive problems and for general behaviour problems were significantly lower for the group treated with fatty acids than for the placebo group. There were significant or almost significant improvements from baseline on seven out of the 14 scales for the fatty acid treatment, compared with none for the placebo. The seven scales showing major improvement with fatty acids were:

- Anxious-Shy ($P = 0.02$)

- Cognitive Problems ($P = 0.02$)

- Psychosomatic ($P = 0.01$)

- Conners' Restless-Impulsive ($P = 0.09$)

- Conners' Emotional Lability ($P = 0.08$)

- Conners' Global Total ($P = 0.05$)

- DSM Inattention ($P = 0.01$)

- DSM Hyperactive-Impulsive ($P = 0.05$), and

- DSM Global Total ($P = 0.05$).

These were dramatic findings showing that intervention with omega-3 and omega-6 fatty acids reduced ADHD symptoms after just three months.

The Durham-Oxford study

To date, the Durham-Oxford study has been the largest clinical trial of fatty acids in ADHD symptoms. Full details of the study are available from the first two papers published from it. One is by Dr Alex Richardson and Dr Paul Montgomery, both from Oxford University, and is called 'The Oxford-Durham study: a randomized, controlled trial of dietary supplementation with fatty acids in children with developmental coordination disorder' and published in the journal *Pediatrics*. The other is by Dr Madeleine Portwood, Dr Shelagh Lowerson (both of Durham County Council) and me. Our paper has the title 'High-eicosapentaenoic acid-containing long-chain polyunsaturated fatty acid supplementation in drug-naïve children with developmental coordination disorder and childhood-occurring dyslexia and attention-deficit hyper-activity disorder symptomatology: a randomised double-blind placebo-controlled clinical trial' and was published in the journal *Prostaglandins, Leukotrienes and Essential Fatty Acids*.

This study had the advantage of using, for the active group, a readily available over-the-counter fatty acid supplement that, at the time the study was carried out, had the highest ratio of

EPA to DHA, in combination with evening primrose oil (which provided GLA). One hundred and ten children aged six to 12 years, attending schools in Durham, England, and who were not receiving any medication were randomly allocated to receive either a high-EPA long-chain polyunsaturated fatty acid supplement or a placebo. These children had a DSM-IV-TR diagnosis of developmental coordination disorder (dyspraxia) and also had ADHD symptoms; you will recall that ADHD and developmental coordination disorder show strong overlap, or comorbidity. The active treatment consisted of the following daily fatty acid doses for three months:

- EPA 558 milligrams

- DHA 174 milligrams

- GLA 60 milligrams.

The placebo used was olive oil.

While the two groups did not differ significantly on standard-ized assessments at the start of the study, after three months the active treatment group showed highly significant improvements in an amazing 12 out of 13 ADHD scales of the Conners' Teacher Rating Scales (Revised: Long Form; Conners, 1997), namely:

- Anxious-Shy ($P = 0.002$)

- Oppositional ($P = 0.01$)

- Cognitive Problems (P less than 0.0005)

- Hyperactivity (P less than 0.0005)

- Social Problems ($P = 0.09$)

- Conners' ADHD Index (P less than 0.0005)

- Conners' Restless-Impulsive (P less than 0.0005)

- Conners' Emotional Lability ($P = 0.02$)

- Conners' Global Total (P less than 0.0005)

- DSM Inattention (P less than 0.0005)

- DSM Hyperactive-Impulsive (P less than 0.0005)

- DSM Global Total (P less than 0.0005).

These are truly amazingly good results, and all from just three months' supplementation with omega-3 and omega-6 fatty acids. In addition, there were significant increases in auditory short-term memory in the active group (P less than 0.0005).

Summary
The paper by Harding, Judah and Gant showed that huge daily dietary supplementation with vitamins, minerals, amino acids and fatty acids was just as effective as methylphenidate in alleviating the symptoms of ADHD. However, I would strongly advise parents of children with ADHD and adults who have the condition *not* to follow such a regime. There is evidence emerging that high doses of certain 'naturally occurring' food ingredients, when taken in supplement form, can potentially be dangerous to our health. One example is vitamin A. I shall say more about this in chapter 7. Another example is the heavy metal chromium, which, like other heavy metals including cadmium, mercury and lead, can be toxic, potentially causing, for instance damage to the kidneys.

We have also seen that evening primrose oil alone is ineffective, as is DHA. In fact, we have seen that DHA has detrimental effects on ADHD symptoms.

The papers by Richardson and Puri, Richardson and Montgomery, and Portwood, Lowerson and Puri, have shown that EPA with evening primrose oil is an effective way of alleviating ADHD symptoms. Unfortunately, the regimes used in these studies included DHA. In chapter 7 I shall outline some of the worrying evidence that indicates that you should *avoid* any supplement that contains DHA. This is not only because DHA has been shown to have detrimental actions on the symptoms of ADHD but, perhaps more worryingly, because of the potential for serious damage to your (or your child's) health from DHA in supplement form.

Fortunately, an over-the-counter supplement is now available to the general public that contains pure EPA, virgin evening primrose oil and absolutely *no* DHA. This is the supplement VegEPA, of which more details (including recommended doses) are given in chapter 7. First, though, we shall look in the next chapter at how standard medication for ADHD compares with fatty acids.

6

Standard medication *versus* fatty acids

At the time of writing, there are three standard medications that are prescribed for the treatment of ADHD:

- Atomoxetine

- Dexamfetamine (dexamphetamine) sulphate, and

- Methylphenidate hydrochloride

Another drug that was used for many years, namely pemoline (trade name Cylert in North America) has been withdrawn from use in many countries because it can cause liver complications. Therefore pemoline will not be discussed in this chapter. Similarly, we shall not deal with other drugs that are occasionally prescribed for children with ADHD but whose primary use lies elsewhere (for instance, tricyclic antidepressants, which are primarily antidepressants; clonidine, which is primarily used for the treatment of high blood pressure, migraine and menopausal flushing; and modafinil, which is primarily used for daytime sleepiness associated with conditions such as narcolepsy, obstructive sleep apnoea syndrome, and chronic shift work).

For each of the three major drugs I shall give the main trade names by which the drug may be more familiar, an outline of the history of its use, the doses recommended, and the side-effects.

Atomoxetine

Trade name
The trade name for atomoxetine is Strattera.

History of use
Atomoxetine was developed by Eli Lilley and Company, one of the world's largest pharmaceutical companies based in Indianapolis in Indiana, USA. Its chemical structure is shown in Figure 14; it is neither a stimulant nor a derivative of amphetamine. It acts by inhibiting, selectively, the reuptake of the neurotransmitter noradrenaline (also known as norepinephrine); to visualize this, just replace dopamine with noradrenaline in Figure 7.

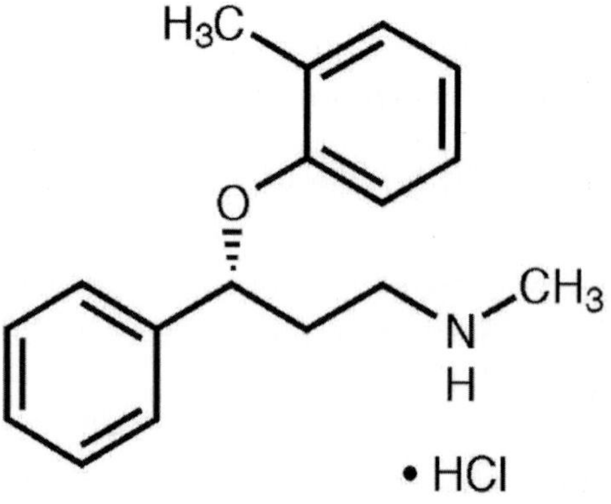

Figure 14. Chemical structure of atomoxetine hydrochloride.

Recommended doses
For children over the age of six years and for adolescents weighing up to 70 kg, the recommended starting dose is 500 micrograms per kilogram body weight per day for the first seven days. The dose of atomoxetine can then be increased according to clinical response up to a maintenance level of 1.2 milligrams per kilogram body weight per day. The maximum dose in this age group is 1.8 milligrams per kilogram body weight per day.

For adolescents weighing more than 70 kg and for adult patients, the recommended starting dose is 40 milligrams per day for the first seven days. The dose of atomoxetine can then be increased according to clinical response up to a maintenance level of 80 milligrams per day. The maximum dose in this age group is 100 milligrams per day.

The total dose may be taken as either one single dose in the morning or else as two divided doses. If taken as two divided doses, the last dose should be taken no later than early evening.

Benefits

Atomoxetine has been found to be better than placebo in alleviating ADHD symptoms in both children and adults.

Side-effects

You may recall that in Chapter 2 I quoted an article from the *Daily Telegraph*, from 2005, which explained that there is a risk of serious liver damage in children who take atomoxetine. As mentioned in the article, if you or your child takes this drug, the signs of liver damage to look out for include:

- Itchy skin

- Dark urine

- Abdominal tenderness

- Jaundice, and

- Unexplained 'flu-like symptoms.

Other side-effects associated with taking atomoxetine include:

- Loss of appetite

- Dry mouth

- Nausea

- Vomiting

- Abdominal pain

- Constipation

- Dyspepsia

- Flatulence

- Palpitations

- Increased heart rate

- Increased blood pressure

- Postural hypotension – in which the patient feels faint on getting up, as if their blood is being drained from their brain; it is similar to the feeling that a normal (unmedicated) person might experience on getting up suddenly after taking a very warm bath

- Hot flushes

- Sleep disturbance

- Dizziness

- Headache

- Fatigue

- Lethargy

- Depression

- Anxiety

- Tremor – shaking of the hands, for example

- Rigors – chills (shivering)

- Retention of urine

- Inflammation of the prostate gland (in males)

- Sexual problems (in adult patients)

- Menstrual disturbances (in menstruating female patients)

- Enlargement of the pupils of the eyes (known as mydriasis)

- Inflammation of the conjunctiva of the eye; the conjunctiva is the thin transparent outer covering of the 'whites' of the eyes

- Inflammation of the skin

- Itching

- Rashes, and

- Sweating.

A less common side-effect associated with atomoxetine treatment is unusually cold hands and feet.

Dexamfetamine

Trade name

The trade name for dexamfetamine (dexamphetamine) sulphate in the United Kingdom is Dexedrine (manufactured by Celltech).

In the United States, dexamfetamine is available in the following preparations:

- Adderall

- Desoxyn

- Desoxyn Gradumet

- Dexedrine

• Dexedrine Spansule

• DextroStat.

In Canada, Dexedrine and Dexedrine Spansule are the main brand names used.

History of use

The history of the use of dexamfetamine (amphetamines) in childhood ADHD has been detailed earlier in this book, in Chapter 4 (see pages 63–70). In summary, it was found by chance to improve attention and hyperactivity in children with ADHD when given to them as a treatment for headaches after they had been subjected to an invasive brain scanning procedure. Subsequent research to investigate why it helps ADHD symptoms has linked its action to problems with the neurotransmitter dopamine but underlying cause and effect remain obscure.

The chemical structure of amphetamine (in a non-sulphated version) has been given in Figure 6.

Recommended doses

For children over the age of six years the daily dose is 5 to 10 milligrams. This can be increased if necessary by 5 milligrams at intervals of one week up to a maximum of 20 milligrams per day. Some doctors sometimes increase the dose to a maximum of 40 milligrams daily in older children.

Benefits

As already mentioned, Dr Charles Bradley was the first to discover that amphetamines can alleviate ADHD symptoms.

Side-effects

The first thing to note is that dexamfetamine should not be taken by anyone who suffers from any of the following conditions:

• Cardiovascular disease – including moderate to severe high blood pressure

- Excitable states or states of agitation

- Hyperthyroidism (overactive thyroid)

- A history of having abused alcohol or illicit drugs, or

- Glaucoma (increased pressure of the fluid in the eye, leading eventually to blindness if untreated).

In addition, dexamfetamine should be avoided by anyone who is pregnant or who is breast-feeding.

Patients who take dexamfetamine may find that their ability to carry out skilled tasks is reduced. It is probably better not to drive, if you are an adult, on this medication. Also, you should really avoid alcohol, as this may interact with the drug.

The more common side-effects associated with dexamfetamine include:

- Insomnia – this is one reason why some drug abusers take amphetamines in the first place, as 'uppers' that will keep them awake

- Restlessness

- Irritability

- Excitability

- Nervousness

- Night terrors

- Euphoria – again, this is a reason why amphetamines are abused, for the 'high' that can be experienced with their use

- Tremor – shaking of the hands, for example

- Dizziness

- Headache

- Convulsions – if there is a history of epilepsy and seizures occur, then the dexamfetamine treatment should be discontinued

- Addiction (to amphetamines)

- Psychosis – the effects can be almost indistinguishable from some types of schizophrenia, at least initially

- Anorexia (loss of appetite)

- Gut problems

- Retarded growth in children – because of this side-effect, the child's growth progress should be regularly monitored by the prescribing doctor

- Dry mouth

- Sweating

- Increased heart rate

- The pain of angina

- Palpitations

- Increased blood pressure – patients taking dexamfetamine should have their blood pressure monitored regularly

- Visual problems, and

- A dangerous heart condition called cardiomyopathy, in which the muscle of the heart becomes inflamed and no longer works as efficiently as before; cardiomyopathy can occur after long-term use of dexamfetamine.

In addition, dexamfetamine can provoke the occurrence of the following movement problems in people who are predisposed to them:

- 'Choreoathetoid movements' – the writhing, 'dancing' movements of the limbs seen, for example, in Huntington's chorea (Huntington's disease)

- Tics

- Tourette syndrome.

Methylphenidate

Trade Name
Methylphenidate has a number of trade names. The most common are Ritalin (manufactured by Cephalon) and Concerta XL (a slow-release form manufactured by Janssen-Cilag).

History of use
Methylphenidate is an artificial compound whose synthesis in the laboratory was first described in 1944. As shown in Figures 1 and 2 the production of methylphnidate and its use in the USA increased dramatically during the 1990s. Its use in other countries also increased during that decade. Its chemical structure is shown in Figure 15. In the 1960s, the first reports appeared of addiction to methylphenidate.

Recommended doses
For children over the age of six years the initial dose is 5 milligrams once to twice daily. This can be increased if necessary by 5 to 10 milligrams at intervals of one week up to a maximum of 60 milligrams per day; a dose this high should not all be taken at once each day, but divided into two or more doses. If there is no beneficial clinical response within one month, then treatment with methylphenidate should be discontinued. It is also recommended that treatment with methylphenidate should be suspended from time to time in order to have an opportunity to assess the child's physical well-being. It is also recommended that the drug should be finally discontinued during or soon after puberty.

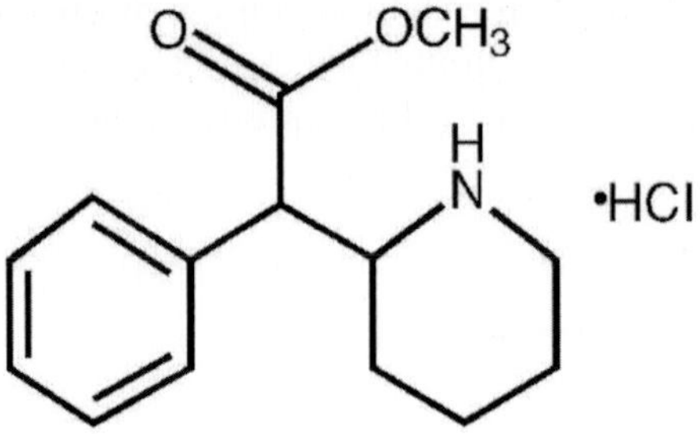

Figure 15. Chemical structure of methylphenidate hydrochloride.

Sometimes the effect of methylphenidate wears off in the evening, with the child showing rebound hyperactivity then. If this keeps occurring, then the doctor may prescribe the child a bedtime dose.

Benefits
Methylphenidate has been found to be better than placebo in alleviating ADHD symptoms in children.

Side-effects
As for dexamfetamine, methylphenidate should not be taken by anyone who suffers from any of the following conditions:

- Cardiovascular disease – including moderate to severe high blood pressure

- Excitable states or states of agitation

- Hyperthyroidism

- A history of having abused alcohol or illicit drugs

- Glaucoma (increased pressure of the fluid in the eye, leading eventually to blindness if untreated).

Similarly, methylphenidate should be avoided by anyone who is pregnant or who is breast-feeding. Patients who take methylphenidate may find that their ability to carry out skilled tasks is reduced. It is probably better not to drive if you are an adult on this medication. Also, you should really avoid alcohol, as this may interact with the drug.

The more common side-effects associated with methyl-phenidate include:

- Insomnia and other sleep disturbances

- Depression

- Confusion

- Restlessness

- Irritability

- Excitability

- Nervousness

- Night terrors

- Euphoria

- Tremor – shaking of the hands, for example

- Rashes

- Itching

- Urticaria – hives or nettlerash

- Dizziness

- Headache

- Fever

- Convulsions – if there is a history of epilepsy, and seizures occur, then the methylphenidate treatment should be discontinued

- Addiction (to methylphenidate)

- Psychosis – the effects can be almost indistinguishable from some types of schizophrenia, at least initially

- Arthralgia (joint pains)

- Loss of appetite

- Alopecia – loss of hair on scalp (balding)

- Gut problems

- Retarded growth in children – because of this side-effect, the child's growth progress should be regularly monitored by the prescribing doctor

- Dry mouth

- Sweating

- Exfoliative dermatitis, a skin condition in which there is a reddening scaly inflammation of much, if not all, the skin; it can be fatal

- Erythema multiforme, which is an allergic reaction of the skin and/or mucous membranes (such as the lips); severe cases require treatment in hospital (in the case of very severe cases, in an intensive care unit or burns unit)

- Increased heart rate

- The pain of angina

- Palpitations

- Increased blood pressure – patients taking methylphenidate should have their blood pressure monitored regularly

- Visual problems

- Cardiomyopathy – see under dexamfetamine (page 134)

- Thrombocytopenic purpura, in which the body's immune system attacks its own platelets in the blood

- Thrombocytopenia, in which there is a reduction in the number of platelets in the blood

- Leucopenia, in which there is a reduction in the number of white blood cells circulating in the blood stream; this can have a negative effect on the immune system

- Urinary problems.

As with dexamfetamine, methylphenidate can provoke the following movement problems in those who are predisposed to them:

- Choreoathetoid movements (involuntary dance-like movements)

- Tics, and

- Tourette syndrome.

Rare side-effects of methylphenidate include:

- Liver damage

- Muscle cramps, and

- Cerebral arteritis, in which there is inflammation of an artery in the brain.

Fatty acids

In contrast to the conventional drugs mentioned above, a fatty acid preparation that consists of a combination of virgin evening primrose oil and pure EPA (that is, with *no* DHA present), is not only safe to take, but has additional benefits besides alleviating symptoms of ADHD. In the next chapter (chapter 7) I shall explain why the evening primrose oil component is so good for us, and why virgin evening primrose oil is even more beneficial than the ordinary refined type. I shall also explain the importance of avoiding any supplements that contain DHA.

Trade names and history of use

Since the first fatty acid study in ADHD (by Dr Richardson and me) was published in 2002, there has been progressive development of fatty acid preparations that, step-by-step, approach the ideal combination of pure EPA, virgin evening primrose oil and zero DHA. At the time that the 2002 study was being carried out, one of the preparations that was closest to this ideal was a product called Efalex Marine or Efamarine (then manufactured by Efamol). This has a small amount of EPA, and rather a lot of DHA. By 2002, the nearest preparation to the ideal formulation was one called eye q (manufactured by Equazen), which unfortunately still contains a fair level of DHA. In 2004 a preparation became available that contains exactly the ideal formulation, namely pure EPA, virgin evening primrose oil, and zero DHA. This is called VegEPA (manufactured by Igennus), and is my preparation of first choice. At the time of writing, all three preparations are widely available.

Recommended doses

At the end of chapter 7 I shall give the ideal formulation of fatty acids to take for ADHD, together with recommended doses. In chapter 8, I shall detail those vitamins and minerals that help the body use these fatty acids efficiently.

Benefits and side-effects

The side-effects of taking the ideal fatty acid preparation are essentially beneficial ones. In chapter 9 I shall describe some of the health benefits of taking a combination of pure EPA and virgin evening primrose oil daily (over and above the benefits in respect of ADHD).

7

How to take fatty acids

Having decided to take omega-3 and omega-6 fatty acids as a natural treatment for ADHD, the patient or parent is faced with a bewildering array of different omega-3 and/or omega-6 preparations, some of which contain concentrated fish oils (for the omega-3), and some of which contain evening primrose oil or starflower oil (for the omega-6). Then there are some so-called experts who claim that all you need to do is eat more oily fish. The aim of this chapter is to help you understand these issues better. With such understanding comes great clarity – by the end of this chapter you will find that you can see right through the forest of competing claims and counter-claims. You will have a clear understanding of the thought processes that have guided me into choosing a unique omega-3 and omega-6 fatty acid supplement that is delivering excellent results in clinical practice, and you will have a sound basis for judging any new product that comes on to the market.

Evening primrose oil

What is evening primrose oil?

Evening primrose oil is extracted from the seeds of the evening primrose plant (latin name, *Oenothera biennis*). This is a wild-flower found growing naturally in Europe, North America, and parts of Asia. Its seeds have been used for centuries by American

Indians. The common name evening primrose derives from the fact that the plant has pale yellow flowers which open in the evening.

Oil extracted from the seeds of the evening primrose plant are rich in the omega-6 long-chain polyunsaturated fatty acid GLA (gamma-linolenic acid). You will recall from the previous chapter that our cells should, in theory, be able to produce GLA from the dietary precursor LA (linoleic acid), so long as the enzyme delta-6-desaturase is functioning properly.

The person who was probably most responsible for bringing evening primrose oil into popular use was the late Professor David Horrobin, who helped set up the company Efamol Ltd and launched the evening primrose oil-based product Efamol. More on the history of evening primrose oil can be found in the excellent short book by Judy Graham, called *Evening Primrose Oil: Its Remarkable Properties and its Use in the Treatment of a Wide Range of Conditions*, first published in 1984.

Benefits

As we saw in chapter 5, taking GLA bypasses any blocks that may be disrupting the action of the enzyme delta-6-desaturase. If you take GLA rather than relying on your body to make it from LA, you will allow your cells and tissues to produce adequate amounts of DGLA (dihomo-gamma-linolenic acid) and AA (arachidonic acid), which in turn are used to form various families of the important, health-promoting eicosanoids (see page 83). Some of the benefits that have been attributed to taking GLA in the form of evening primrose oil include:

- Improvement in certain skin conditions

- Improvement of the nails

- Improvement of the skin generally

- Improvement in premenstrual syndrome (PMS, or pre-menstrual tension or PMT)

- Improvement in breast pain (mastalgia), and

- Improvement in nerve damage in diabetes mellitus.

Why virgin?

Rather than suggest that my patients (or, in the case of children, their parents) go out and buy the cheapest evening primrose oil capsules they can find, I recommend that they take a special form of evening primrose oil, known as virgin evening primrose oil. Why?

Ordinary evening primrose oil preparations are made by processing the seed oil at relatively high temperatures and in other ways that remove some of the beneficial properties from the oil. In the same way that modern industrial processing of wheat grains strips away many nutritious and important substances (such as fibre, certain vitamins and minerals) to leave the pale, far less tasty, constipating 'food' we know as white flour, so modern industrial processing of evening primrose oil strips away much of the goodness and rich full flavour of the natural oil to leave what is, in essence, a pale imitation. To carry the analogy further, whereas most commercially available evening primrose oil preparations are like white flour, virgin (non-raffinated, cold-pressed) evening primrose oil is like wholemeal flour, complete with the goodness still intact.

In 2004 I published a paper entitled 'The clinical advantages of cold-pressed non-raffinated evening primrose oil over refined preparations.' For the purposes of this study, I started by looking at two common commercially available over-the-counter sets of capsules of evening primrose oil. On syringing out the contents of these capsules, I saw a pale, insipid-coloured (non-virgin, refined) evening primrose oil. However, I had a vial of a third evening primrose oil preparation available to me. This was of virgin evening primrose oil (exactly as is now contained in the supplement VegEPA). Instead of the pale, straw-coloured liquid I was used to, the virgin evening primrose oil was a deep rich green colour.

In 2002, Matthias Hamburger and his colleagues from the Institute of Pharmacy, Friedrich-Schiller-University Jena, in Jena and the Institute of Pharmacy, Humboldt-University Berlin, in Berlin, published a paper in the *Journal of Agricultural and Food Chemistry* in which they showed that virgin (cold-pressed, non-raffinated) evening primrose oil is rich in a group of compounds known as triterpines. In contrast, they reported that commercial samples of (non-virgin) evening primrose oil contained only traces of triterpines. Triterpines are naturally occurring compounds that help the body mop up dangerous 'free radicals', that enable our white blood cells to function better, and that help reduce the pain of arthritic joints.

Omega-3 fatty acids

Why not just eat more fish?
You have seen why I favour virgin evening primrose oil as the source of the omega-6 fatty acid GLA (gamma-linolenic acid). When it comes to the omega-3 side of the equation, as I explained in Chapter 5, I would strongly favour taking EPA. However, there is a school of thought that argues that patients can obtain the EPA they need just by eating more fish. In principle, it is true that fish, particularly oily fish such as salmon, trout, herrings, tuna, mackerel and sardines, are a good source of EPA. There are, though, at least two disadvantages to this approach.

First, in order to obtain a high enough quantity of EPA, you would have to eat a very large amount of fish each day. I tend to start my adult ADHD patients on a dose of omega-3 and omega-6 fatty acid supplement that delivers over 2,000 milligrams EPA daily. In order to obtain that from fish, my patients would have to consume around 400 grams of fresh tuna or trout each day, or around 200 grams of mackerel.

The second disadvantage is even more compelling. Humans have been busy polluting the rivers, seas and oceans of the world with toxins such as heavy metals (like lead, mercury and cadmium), dioxins (a generic term which covers polychlorinated dibenzo-p-dioxins and dibenzofurans) and PCBs (polychlorinated biphenyls). Heavy metals such as mercury and cadmium can be dangerous to the body, including the brain, while dioxins and PCBs have been linked to illnesses such as cancer. Furthermore, although there may be relatively low concentrations of these pollutants in seawater, they are concentrated by each successively higher level of the food chain. So, by the time top marine predators in the food chain such as trout and salmon are reached, the concentrations of these dangerous chemicals may have reached levels that are a million times greater than in the surrounding seawater.

What about ordinary fish oil capsules?

Ordinary fish oil suffers from the same problems as the ones we have just mentioned in relation to the risk from pollutants such as lead, mercury, cadmium, dioxins and PCBs. In fact, there are at least three reasons why the situation is even worse for fish oil than it is for ordinary fish in the diet.

First, many of the harmful pollutants that are concentrated in the bodies of fish, such as dioxins and PCBs, are highly fat-soluble. This means that they are even more concentrated in fish oils (which, by definition, are oils and therefore fatty).

Second, we need to consider how fish oils tend to be extracted in industrial quantities from the bodies of fish. One method often used in industry is simply to squeeze the livers of the fish, and use the liver oil thereby produced. A common example is cod liver oil, which has a good deal of EPA in it, and is extracted, unsurprisingly, from the livers of cod. A major problem with this process is that in vertebrates such as fish (and, indeed, us), the liver is the main organ used for the detoxification of the blood. So, the liver oils can offer an even more concentrated concoction of dangerous pollutants. Another commonly used method is not to squeeze just the liver of the fish, but instead to squeeze the whole body of the fish, and collect the oil that comes out of the back passage. Needless to say, the alimentary tract is a very good source of the poisons that the vertebrate body may wish to get rid of.

The third reason is that fish oil is rich in vitamin A. Healthy adults tend to have large stores of this vitamin in their livers. If taken in excessive quantities, vitamin A is toxic, and can even be fatal. To obtain one to two grams of EPA daily, the amount of ordinary fish oil that needs to be taken could be dangerous, because the daily intake of vitamin A could easily reach the toxic range. (Note that it is also possible to become vitamin A toxic from vegetables that contain the vitamin A precursor beta-carotene. For instance, there was a case in the 1990s of a man in Britain who used to drink large amounts of carrot juice several times daily, every day. Eventually, the toxic levels of vitamin A he was building up in his liver caused irreparable damage to this organ. He died from the high intake of vitamin A. Another reason for my recommending VegEPA over other supplements is that it is completely free of vitamin A.)

The fourth reason for not taking fish oil as a supplement is that, in addition to containing EPA, it also contains DHA. I shall now explain why any supplement containing DHA should be avoided.

DHA

Why is a DHA-free supplement better?

With one exception, at the time of writing this book all the EPA-containing supplements available to the general public also contain the omega-3 long-chain polyunsaturated fatty acid DHA (docosahexaenoic acid). As an illustration, in Table 1, I have listed for supplements currently available in the UK the relative amounts of EPA and DHA that their manufacturers ascribe to them.

So why do some of the leading *researchers* in the field of lipids refuse to take supplements that contain DHA? There are several reasons.

The first reason we shall look at is a practical one. If a supplement contains both EPA and DHA, then it is likely that it is simply fish oil. The oil extracted from oily fish (whether from the liver or squeezed through the alimentary tract) tends to be rich in both EPA and DHA. But we have just seen why fish oil can be dangerous to our health, if it contains heavy metals and poisonous fat-soluble

Table 1. Relative levels of EPA and DHA in readily available fatty acid preparations (figures based on those published by manufacturers)

Preparation	EPA (mg) per capsule	DHA (mg) per capsule	Ratio of EPA to DHA
Efamarine	17	11	1.5
eye q	93	29	3.2
Maxepa	170	115	1.5
VegEPA	280	0	Infinity

pollutants such as dioxins and PCBs. When a mass-produced fish oil preparation contains both EPA and DHA, it is far cheaper to make it by simply packing fish oil, than for companies carefully to extract pure EPA and pure DHA and then put them together without any other components of the fish oil (including the pollutants). In contrast, in the case of the one product available to the general public that contains virgin evening primrose oil combined with EPA but no DHA whatsoever (namely, VegEPA), just ultra-pure EPA has been extracted from the fish oil, using a cold extraction method, and everything else in the fish oil, including the DHA and the pollutants, has been discarded. It is rather like taking ordinary river water, and distilling off and collecting ultra-pure water from it. This water would be extremely safe to drink and would contain no pollutants. To follow through this analogy, the ultra-pure EPA would be to ordinary fish oil as ultra-pure water would be to ordinary river water.

The second reason for avoiding supplements that contain DHA will almost certainly already have occurred to you when you were reading Chapter 5. You will recall from that chapter that studies of children with ADHD in which DHA was used predominantly or solely as the long-chain polyunsaturated fatty acid supplement have shown that DHA is no better than placebo. In fact, we saw that careful analysis of the results of these studies showed that children with ADHD who received DHA actually fared *worse* than the corresponding placebo groups.

A third reason why we should avoid supplements that contain DHA is that some of the leading researchers in the field have come to the conclusion that when ingested, the type of DHA that comes in supplements (as opposed to occurring naturally in food) tends to inhibit many of the beneficial actions of EPA. (You may recall from earlier in this book how EPA is a direct precursor of many families of eicosanoids, and how it can also kill harmful viruses and also form natural sleep mediators that promote deep, refreshing sleep.) The reason for this is not yet known but is under investigation.

As if these arguments against DHA were not enough, yet another reason is emerging for avoiding DHA in supplement form. In June 2004, Dr Thorlaksdottir, from the Department of Biochemistry and Molecular Biology, School of Medicine, University of Iceland, together with colleagues from other departments and from the Icelandic Cancer Society, presented some new results from a study that they had just completed but not yet published in a scientific or medical journal. They looked at the number of breaks in the DNA (deoxyribonucleic acid) molecules of the nuclei of certain white blood cells called peripheral blood mononuclear cells and the relationship between the number of these DNA breaks and levels of fatty acids.

DNA makes up the genes and chromosomes of cells. It is important that DNA strands do not break, as this can mean that the cell might mutate. Such mutation in turn means there might be a risk of cancer developing.

Dr Thorlaksdottir and her colleagues looked at these DNA breaks in 98 healthy women, whose average age was 46 years. A wide range of DNA damage was found in the women. Dr Thorlaksdottir and her colleagues also looked at levels of many different fatty acids, including omega-3 and omega-6 fatty acids, saturated fatty acids and monounsaturated fatty acids in the membranes of red blood cells. In the case of just two of these fatty acids, there was a positive correlation (or association) between the level of the fatty acid and the amount of DNA damage. The two fatty acids were DHA and linoleic acid (LA). The higher the level of either DHA or LA in red blood cell membranes, the greater the amount of DNA damage measured in the white blood cells. (There were no such statistically significant associations between DNA damage and DGLA, AA or EPA.) Fortunately, we do not have to worry too much about linoleic acid, because it is 'compartmentalized' soon after we absorb it – very little if any can be detected in the brain, even when it is being regularly consumed. Alas, the same is not true for DHA.

The conclusion that Dr Thorlaksdottir and her colleagues from the University of Iceland and the Icelandic Cancer Society came to was that:

> These data suggest that dietary linoleic acid and DHA may be positively associated with DNA damage.

Dr Thorlaksdottir and her colleagues wondered if the mechanism of the DNA damage was the result of the way in which some fatty acids are prone to becoming oxidized, and that this oxidative damage might result in products (such as free radicals) that in turn could cause DNA damage. (Incidentally, this is another reason why the triterpines in virgin evening primrose oil – but not in ordinary processed evening primrose oil – are so helpful, as they can, as it were, mop up free radicals.)

Avoiding DHA from supplements is easy, though not cheap relative to straightforward fish oil supplements, as extracting EPA without DHA from fish oil is a complicated process; to obtain EPA alone you can just take the DHA-free supplement VegEPA.

Although at the time of writing Dr Thorlaksdottir and her colleagues had not yet published their work formally in a journal, they did manage to present their study in abstract form at a conference (see the References section at the end of this book). Worryingly, their abstract began with the following sentence:

> DNA modification is believed to be an important step in carcinogenesis [that is, the development of cancer].

But don't we need DHA?

Sometimes, when I explain to patients the virtues of taking a supplement that contains a combination of virgin evening primrose oil and ultra-pure EPA, which crucially is completely DHA-free, they worry about the fact that they have read articles stating that we need DHA. Will they not end up being deficient in DHA, they wonder.

It is perfectly true that DHA is useful to the body – but only in a limited way. If you re-read part of Chapter 5 (see page 83), you will recall that the main function of DHA in the body is a structural one. It helps form the correct, flexible, structure of the membranes that bound both cells and the organelles inside cells. If you take ultra-pure EPA (without any DHA) then your body can readily make DHA as and when it is needed, in just the right places where it is required, from the EPA you have taken. Just glance at Figure 13 again to see how the body can do this.

(In re-examining Figure 13, you will notice that, to make DHA from EPA, the problematic enzyme delta-6-desaturase is needed once again. Although it is one of the enzymes used here, there are several reasons why it can help the body at this stage in the fatty acid chain while being inhibited at the crucial earlier stage. First, the amounts of DHA needed are very low so only a small amount of the enzyme is needed. Second, by taking large amounts of EPA, the 'substrate binding site' (the place on the enzyme that locks on to the fatty acids it is helping to break down) on the delta-6-desaturase enzyme is competitively 'saturated' with the EPA derivative; this means that available delta-6-desturase is used for this process to the exclusion of others. Third, if a virus is (partly) responsible for blocking the enzyme, then the EPA will inhibit that inhibition, if you see what I mean! Finally, fourth, I hope you will, in addition to taking EPA, also take on board my advice about a change in diet and the addition, if necessary, of cofactors, which will also help.)

What about flaxseed oil?

There is an argument that people who need more EPA, including those who suffer from ADHD, can get all they need from flaxseed oil, particularly if they are vegetarian and therefore unable to eat fish (The oil is derived from the seeds of the flax plant.) This is, in my view, a disingenuous argument. The omega-3 fatty acid that flaxseed oil provides is ALA (alpha-linolenic acid). Looking again at Figure 13, you will see that ALA is the dietary short-chain precursor of all the long-chain omega-3 fatty acids, including EPA. But to get anywhere near EPA down the omega-3 chain, first the ALA has to be converted into another fatty acid (called octade-catetraenoic acid), which involves the enzyme delta-6-desaturase. However, you will recall that this enzyme can be blocked by various factors, and is probably blocked in most cases of ADHD. Since we are attempting to bypass this block in ADHD, it does not make sense to take flaxseed oil.

The ideal formulation

From the information presented in this chapter, we can see that the perfect omega-3 and omega-6 fatty acid formulation to take would be one that contains a combination of:

- Virgin evening primrose oil (as opposed to ordinary refined evening primrose oil that is lacking in triter-pines that scavenge free radicals)

- Pure EPA, and

- Zero DHA.

At the time of writing, there is just one clinically-tested supplement available to the general public that provides this ideal combination. This is VegEPA, which is available at www.vegepa.com, or from the address or telephone number given in the section on Useful names and addresses at the end of the book. Each VegEPA capsule contains:

- 100 milligrams virgin evening primrose oil

- 280 milligrams pure EPA

- Zero DHA.

As you would expect from the discussion earlier, the capsules are free of any pollutants, and free of vitamin A.

Dose

VegEPA is perfectly safe for almost everyone. The one possible exception is people who have a bleeding disorder or who are on blood thinning agents (anticoagulant medication) such as warfarin tablets or heparin injections. Even in these cases, it is usually safe to take a reduced dose of the fatty acid supplement, but you should consult your doctor first.

For children with ADHD between the ages of five and 12 years, the recommended dose is two VegEPA capsules daily. These can be taken together in the morning or evening, or as one capsule twice daily. If a child does not like swallowing large capsules, the capsules can be snipped in two and the contents added to a drink or food (such as yoghurt).

For children with ADHD aged between 12 and 16 years, the daily dose is four VegEPA capsules. Again, these can be taken together or in divided doses (say, two twice daily), preferably with food.

Adult ADHD sufferers should take eight capsules daily, preferably as four capsules twice daily with food.

8

The vitamin and mineral cofactors

What are cofactors?

You may have noticed in the preceding chapters that when you take a fatty acid supplement as a natural treatment for ADHD, there are many enzymes involved in the reactions that have to take place in the body. Some of these are shown in Box 6:

Box 6. Enzymes involved in fatty acid metabolism

- The conversion of the omega-6 fatty acid GLA into DGLA (dihomo-gamma-linolenic acid). (The enzyme involved is called *elongase*.)

- The conversion of the omega-6 fatty acid DGLA into AA (arachidonic acid). (The enzyme involved is called *delta-5-desaturase* – not to be confused with *delta-6-desaturase*.)

- The conversion of DGLA and AA into different families of eicosanoids.

- The conversion of the omega-3 fatty acid EPA into docosapentaenoic acid (using the enzyme *elongase*). Then the conversion of docosapentaenoic acid into tetracosapen-taenoic acid (using the enzyme *elongase*). Then the conversion of tetracosapentaenoic acid into tetrahexaenoic acid (using the enzyme *delta-6-desaturase*, which is unlikely to be inhibited at this later stage in the fatty acid chain (see page 148)). Then the conversion of tetrahexaenoic acid into DHA (using *beta-oxidation*).

> • The conversion of EPA into different families of eicosanoids.
>
> • The conversion of EPA into interferons. (The enzymes involved include *cyclo-oxygenase* and *lipo-oxygenase*.)

The details in the above list are not too important for our purposes. Instead, I want to draw your attention to the many enzymes involved. In fact, I have only skimmed the surface in this respect; there are many more. For all these enzymes and enzyme-mediated conversions to function properly, small amounts of certain vitamins and minerals need to be present in the body. These are known as 'cofactors', and their absence makes it difficult for all the reactions to take place properly. So we need to make sure we are not deficient in any of these cofactors.

The most important cofactors

The main vitamins that we need are:

- Folic acid

- Vitamin B_{12}

- Vitamin B_6

- Niacin

- Biotin, and

- Vitamin C.

These are all B vitamins, apart from the last one (vitamin C). The main minerals (actually 'trace elements') we need are:

- Zinc

- Selenium, and

- Magnesium.

If we are deficient in these vitamins, it may be because we are not eating the right foods that are rich in them; another reason may be that we are not absorbing the food properly (malabsorption). If you believe that you have (or your child has) an illness that is causing you not to absorb your food properly, then you should see your doctor. Here, I shall assume that you can absorb your intake of these B vitamins, vitamin C, and trace elements.

In general, it is better to obtain these cofactors naturally, in your diet. This means you need to know which foods are rich in each cofactor. This chapter will give you this information. For those of you who prefer to 'play safe' and take vitamin and mineral supplements, I have included a brief section that deals with this at the end of this chapter.

You will see I have given the recommended daily intake levels (dietary reference values) for these vitamins and minerals, where these are known, for adults and, in selected cases, for young children aged between four and six years. (I have included these where they are known; there are no recommended daily intake levels for some of the cofactors.) The corresponding values for older children and adolescents are intermediate between the doses for young children and those for adults.

The B vitamins

Folic acid, vitamin B_{12}, vitamin B_6, niacin and biotin are all B vitamins. They are water-soluble. This means they can leach into cooking water and excessive intake from food is rarely dangerous because you can excrete the B vitamins from your body in your urine.

Folic acid

Folic acid is also known as folate and folacin. One of its chemical names is pteroylmonoglutamic acid. Unlike the other B vitamins, folic acid can actually be stored in the liver, and so it is not quite so important to maintain a regular intake of this vitamin. In the United Kingdom, the adult recommended intake is 200 micrograms per day. For children aged between four and six years, the recommended intake is 100 micrograms per day. (A microgram is a millionth of a gram. This is a very small amount.)

Good dietary sources of folic acid include:

- Leafy green vegetables

- Green beans

- Peas

- Other pulses (such as beans and lentils)

- Yeast extract

- Mushrooms

- Nuts

- Whole grains

- Liver, and

- Certain fortified breakfast cereals.

With this and the other lists of foods given below for each cofactor, the important thing is to make sure you (or your child) get at least one portion of at least one of the foods in your diet each day. There is really no need to weigh out the food to try to ensure that you (or your child) are eating the recommended intake. For one thing, the recommended intake can vary between different countries. More importantly, in general the body only needs a small amount of these vitamins and minerals every day. If you (or your child) are not deficient to begin with, then so long as you are eating something from each of the lists each day, you should be all right.

For those readers with an interest in medicine, I shall simply note that deficiency in folic acid can cause megaloblastic or macrocytic anaemia, without going into any further details about what this condition is.

Vitamin B_{12}

Vitamin B_{12} consists of a group of molecules which all contain the element cobalt. Collectively they are known as cobalamins, with subtypes including hydroxocobalamin and cyanocobalamin.

Contrary to common belief, not *all* microbes are bad for us. Far from it. Some microbes are actually good for us and can help supply our bodies with certain nutrients. Vitamin B_{12} is an example where this applies.

Although vitamin B_{12} is not of vegetable origin, in general healthy vegetarians should be able to obtain sufficient quantities from microbes that are to be found in their gastrointestinal tract (particularly the intestines and the mouth). Also, microbial contamination of food will deliver vitamin B_{12} to the human body. Yes, a bit of food contamination is not necessarily a bad thing!

Having said that, there is a theoretical risk that strict vegetarians who eat food that has been irradiated to kill all microbes may eventually become deficient. In healthy individuals, there is enough vitamin B_{12} stored in the liver to last for at least three years. In the United Kingdom, the recommended intake for adults is 1.5 micrograms per day; the corresponding figure is 2 micrograms per day in the United States. (This is just one of many examples in which the United States has set a slightly different recommended daily allowance to that set in the United Kingdom.)

Dietary sources of vitamin B_{12} include:

- Meat

- Milk, and

- Contamination of food with micro-organisms, mould, faecal matter, insects or insect droppings.

Although milk is a good source, be aware that the vitamin may be destroyed by boiling or by adding the milk to boiling water when making tea or coffee.

Deficiency in vitamin B_{12} can cause megaloblastic or macrocytic anaemia, and prolonged deficiency can lead to subacute combined degeneration of the spinal cord.

Vitamin B$_6$

Vitamin B$_6$ is available in food in the forms pyridoxine, pyridoxal and pyridoxamine. These three forms of vitamin B$_6$ are all active and can be converted into each other. In the United Kingdom, the recommended daily intake (for adults) is 1.5 micrograms per gram of dietary protein.

Good dietary sources of vitamin B$_6$ include:

- Whole grains

- Cereals

- Leafy green vegetables

- Eggs

- Meat

- Liver

- Fish

- Pulses (beans and peas)

- Fruit, and

- Green beans.

Deficiency is rare but be aware that some medications can interact with vitamin B$_6$ and thereby produce a deficiency; they include: isoniazid, hydralazine, and penicillamine. Deficiency in babies can cause convulsions. Deficiency in adults can lead to anaemia, a smooth and inflamed tongue, lips that are raw with lesions in the corners of the mouth, dermatitis, and fatigue. (Dermatitis is inflammation of the skin. It is essentially the same thing as eczema.)

Niacin

Niacin is also known as nicotinic acid or vitamin B_3. It can be made by the liver from an amino acid called tryptophan; 60 milligrams of dietary tryptophan are converted into 1 milligram of niacin. (One milligram is a thousandth of a gram.) Eggs and cheese are good sources of tryptophan. It tends to be added to many breakfast cereals and to white flour in many countries. (Niacin is lost when wheat is processed to make white flour.) In the United Kingdom, the recommended daily intake for adults is 6.6 milligrams per 1000 kcal dietary energy intake. (One kcal is a kilocalorie, which is one thousand calories. This is a measure of the energy content of food.) For children between the ages of four and six years, the recommended United Kingdom daily intake is 11 milligrams.

Good dietary sources of niacin include:

- Pulses (beans and peas)

- Meat

- Milk

- Nuts

- Liver

- Fish

- Whole grains, and

- Certain fortified breakfast cereals.

Deficiency in niacin can cause pellagra, a condition in which dermatitis, diarrhoea and dementia occur. Niacin deficiency can occur in people who eat almost only maize (for instance, in some parts of Africa), partly because maize is low in tryptophan and partly because the niacin in maize is present in the form niacytin, which is not active biologically in the same way as ordinary niacin. Niacin deficiency can also occur following treatment with the drug isoniazid. Those who eat a diet that contains a very low level of proteins can also become niacin deficient, as can those who suffer from alcoholism and do not eat properly.

Other causes of niacin deficiency include the carcinoid syndrome and phaeochromocytomas. Carcinoid syndrome is a condition in which patients suffer from facial and neck blushing, abdominal pains and watery diarrhoea, which keeps recurring, as well as some heart problems. It can result from a particular type of growth in the bowels, called a carcinoid tumour, which then spreads to the liver. These tumours secrete the transmitter serotonin, which causes the diarrhoea.

Phaeochromocytomas are tumours that arise usually in the adrenal glands. (The adrenal glands are two glands that lie just above the kidneys.) The adrenal glands secrete noradrenaline (also known as norepinephrine) and adrenaline (epinephrine) into the circulation.

Biotin

Biotin is also known as coenzyme R, vitamin H and, originally, the anti-egg white injury factor. In the United Kingdom, the recommended intake for adults is between 10 and 200 micrograms per day, while in the United States the corresponding recommended intake range is between 30 and 100 micrograms per day.

Good dietary sources of biotin include:

- Nuts

- Fruit

- Whole, brown rice

- Yeast

- Cooked eggs

- Cereals, and

- Liver.

Deficiency in biotin can occur in those who eat a lot of raw eggs, owing to the fact that raw egg white contains a protein (avidin) that acts to prevent the absorption of biotin; avidin is destroyed by cooking eggs. If a mother is not well fed, then her breast milk may be very low in biotin, which can cause dermatitis in her baby.

In adults, taking biotin can help rejuvenate the hair follicles. In other words, if you are beginning to lose your hair, sometimes taking biotin can help your hair follicles to start growing thicker hair again. If, in addition, you take a fatty acid supplement that contains virgin evening primrose oil and pure EPA, then you are feeding your hair follicles with excellent nutrients. (One man of my acquaintance started to take the fatty acid supplement that contains virgin evening primrose oil and pure EPA every day. Within eight weeks his hair had started to change from being dry and wiry into a luscious growth. His barber was pleasantly surprised. (Incidentally, his skin also changed. When he started the supplement he could have passed for a sixty-year-old. Now he looks as if he is in his forties.)

Vitamin C

Vitamin C is also known as ascorbic acid or ascorbate and is water-soluble. Unlike most other mammals, unfortunately human bodies cannot make their own vitamin C and so we must obtain this important antioxidant in our diets. In the United Kingdom, the recommended daily intake for adults is 40 milligrams, while the corresponding figure in the United States is 60 milligrams. The late Linus Pauling (winner of two Nobel prizes) recommended much higher doses, although if there is any impairment of kidney function, then a very high dose can lead to the formation of kidney stones. Linus Pauling argued that the government nutrition bodies were being too conservative. By looking at the amount of vitamin C that an average adult gorilla eats each day in the wild, and then extrapolating back to the average human body weight, he suggested that adult humans need well over a gram of this vitamin each day. For children between the ages of four and six years, the recommended United Kingdom daily intake is 30 milligrams.

Good dietary sources of vitamin C include:

- Fruit – such as citrus fruits, fresh strawberries, cantaloupe, pineapples and guava

- Vegetables – such as broccoli, Brussels sprouts, tomatoes, potatoes, spinach, kale, green peppers, cabbage and turnips, and

- Fresh milk.

Vitamin C is easily leached out of vegetables that are being cooked in water. Cooking also oxidizes the vitamin, as does exposure to alkalis or copper. The vitamin C content of potatoes gradually diminishes with storage of this vegetable. Vitamin C deficiency sometimes occurs in infants who are fed boiled milk. Deficiency invitamin C can cause scurvy, which may start with weakness and muscle pains, followed by the more 'classical signs' for which the condition is famous: bleeding gums, teeth becoming loose, wounds not healing properly, and bleeding under the skin. Anaemia is also likely, as vitamin C is needed to help with the absorption of iron from the diet.

The trace elements

Trace elements are mineral elements that are required in 'trace' (barely discernible) amounts in the diet for the maintenance of good health. Zinc, selenium and magnesium are all elements that have to be obtained by dietary means and that act as cofactors for fatty acid metabolism.

Zinc

Zinc can help wound healing, prostate problems and infertility. It can help promote mental alertness. In the United Kingdom, the recommended daily intake for adults is 9.5 milligrams for men and 7 milligrams for women. For children between the ages of four and six years, the recommended United Kingdom daily intake is 6.5 milligrams.

Good dietary sources of zinc include:

- Meat

- Wholegrain products

- Pulses (peas and beans)

- Yeast, and

- Pumpkin seeds.

Clinically, zinc deficiency may cause white spots under the fingernails and poor healing of wounds. With severe zinc deficiency, there may be loss of hair, night blindness, and impaired taste and smell.

Selenium

Selenium acts as an antioxidant in conjunction with vitamin E. It can help return a youthful elasticity to tissues, and alleviate some of the effects of the menopause such as hot flushes. In the United Kingdom, the recommended intake of selenium for adults is 60 micrograms per day.

Good dietary sources of selenium include:

- Meat

- Wholegrain products

- Fish, and

- Vegetables.

In some countries, such as the United States and Canada, the soil is relatively rich in selenium, so that the flour produced there contains sufficient quantities. However, European wheat is rather impoverished in this respect, while the soil in parts of China has very low levels of this trace element.

Severe selenium deficiency can cause a potentially fatal heart disease (cardiomyopathy) known as Keshan disease; this sometime occurs in those parts of China where the population depends on crops grown on selenium deficient soil. It is not known whether there are any direct clinical effects from mild selenium deficiency (other than adverse effects on making fatty acids).

Magnesium

Magnesium occurs as part of the green chlorophyll pigment of plants. It helps promote a healthy cardiovascular system and is involved in calcium metabolism. Its levels in the human body can become depleted by alcohol.

Good dietary sources of magnesium include:

- Vegetables – particularly fresh green vegetables and corn

- Pulses (peas and beans), and

- Fruit – including apples.

A severe deficiency, for example as a result of alcoholism, can cause seizures.

Supplements

It is best to obtain the cofactors (the B vitamins, vitamin C, and the trace elements) from your diet, by ensuring that your daily food intake includes at least one of the foodstuffs from the list for each cofactor. However, you may have a problem adhering to such a regime. As an adult ADHD sufferer you may be too busy to find the time to eat a proper, suitably varied diet. Or you may find that you are sometimes too tired to prepare such meals. In cases like this, it is better to take a supplement rather than miss out altogether on the necessary cofactors.

For the B vitamins, there are vitamin B complex supplements available, while vitamin C supplements (both tablets that are swallowed and tablets and powder preparations that are dissolved in water) can also be readily bought over-the-counter in chemists (pharmacies) and supermarkets. To be on the safe side and make sure you do not miss out on any of these vitamins, you could consider taking a multivitamin supplement. If choosing a multivitamin, you should check that it does deliver all the B vitamins mentioned above. In general, it is a good idea to take just the stated dose. In other words, unless you have carefully researched the doses and know why you want to take a high dose of a certain vitamin, then it is safest to stay within the Recommended Daily Allowances for each vitamin. (Some people are happy to take higher doses of vitamin C, for example, but in such cases they should ensure they do not suffer from kidney disease, as there is a risk in those circumstances of kidney stones being formed.) For children with ADHD, it really is best to change their diet so that it contains the necessary cofactors. If this just is not possible, then only use multivitamin supplements that are specifically made for their age group.

A similar set of considerations applies to choosing supplements of trace elements. Buying multi-mineral supplements that contain zinc, selenium and magnesium is often cheaper than purchasing separate supplements for each of these three trace elements. In the cases of zinc and selenium, I would strongly recommend that you stay within the Recommended Daily Allowances for each trace element. It is possible to suffer from the effects of toxicity if you take too much zinc or selenium daily.

Finally, there are some preparations available that are combined multivitamin and multi-mineral supplements. So long as they contain all the cofactors mentioned in this chapter, then it is absolutely fine to take these at the dose I have given. Again, for children, only use children's preparations that contain smaller doses of these vitamins and trace elements. Recently, two very safe multivitamin/multimineral preparations have become available that contain only the particular cofactors mentioned in this chapter, and only in doses less than the recommended daily allowances. One is called VegeCO, and is specifically for adults. Each VegeCO tablet contains:

Folic Acid	100 micrograms
Vitamin B_{12}	0.75 micrograms
Vitamin B_6	0.5 milligrams
Niacin	6 milligrams
Biotin	10 micrograms
Vitamin C	20 milligrams
Zinc	3.5 milligrams
Selenium	30 micrograms
Magnesium	200 micrograms

It is perfectly safe for an adult to take one VegeCO tablet daily. The other preparation has been designed for children, and is called mini-VegeCO. Each mini-VegeCO tablet contains:

Folic Acid	10 micrograms
Vitamin B_{12}	0.075 micrograms
Vitamin B_6	0.05 milligrams
Niacin	0.6 milligrams
Biotin	1 microgram
Vitamin C	2 milligrams
Zinc	0.35 milligrams
Selenium	3 micrograms
Magnesium	20 micrograms

It is perfectly safe for children aged between six and 12 years to take one mini-VegeCO tablet daily. Children aged over 12 years can safely take two mini-VegeCO tablets daily. (The outer shell of VegeCO and mini-VegeCO is vegetarian and so is free of gelatine. Instead it is made from tapioca, which is a cassava root starch.)

9

Other benefits from taking fatty acids

There are a number of known side-effects from taking an omega-3 and omega-6 fatty acid supplement but none that are seriously negative and many that are wholly beneficial. I shall examine them in this chapter.

The only side-effect that might be regarded as adverse is a slight loosening of the bowel contents. This may occur with an adult dose of eight VegEPA capsules daily. However, this is actually a good thing because if the passage of material speeds up in your gut, then there is less time for toxins to be absorbed into your system. Some scientists think that as a result you might reduce your risks of getting bowel cancer. Other ways of doing this include ensuring you have a lot of fibre in your diet. A good way to do this is to choose unrefined products over refined products. For example, wholemeal flour and bread are better than white flour and bread. Again, brown rice is better than white rice.

The other 'side-effects' of a supplement containing pure EPA and virgin evening primrose oil are also good for us. In fact, they are so beneficial that, in general, almost everyone can benefit from taking such a supplement daily (albeit at a lower dose of, say, four VegEPA capsules daily for adults who do not suffer from ADHD; two capsules daily for those aged 12 to 16 years, and one capsule daily between the ages of five and 12 years). The only slight caution is in respect of those who are taking a blood-thinning drug such as warfarin or heparin – this is explained on page 173 in the section called 'Cardiovascular system'. In fact, although I have never suffered from ADHD, I take eight capsules daily – four each morning and four each evening, with food which helps with their digestion but is not essential.

Mood and combating depression

Pure EPA (without any DHA) acts as a powerful, yet safe, mood elevating substance. In fact, so good is pure EPA in doing this that it has actually been found to have antidepressant actions in severe depression. The evidence for this has been outlined in Chapter 5.

Sleep

As I mentioned in Chapter 5, EPA is converted into natural sleep mediators. After a few days to a few weeks of taking pure EPA (without any DHA), even people who do not suffer from ADHD find that they experience sleep that is much deeper and much more refreshing than they might be used to. From personal experience, the best description I can think of to describe just how pleasant this sleep is (and I had never had problems sleeping during my adult life prior to starting to take EPA) is a verse from the Wisdom literature to be found in the Bible in Proverbs chapter 3 verse 24:

> Yea, thou shalt lie down,
> And thy sleep shall be sweet.

Energy

Regular intake of an omega-3 and omega-6 fatty acid supplement is associated with increased energy levels. Part of this may be by virtue of the improved more refreshing sleep that people enjoy. There are also other reasons for the improved energy, including the fact that the body's cells and tissues are now able to make sufficient quantities of different eicosanoid families (see Chapter 5) from virgin evening primrose oil and pure EPA. The body now has at its disposal a full complement of stress-busting substances within the context of an immune system that is geared up and finely tuned.

Concentration, reading and thinking

Whether or not a person is suffering from ADHD to begin with, they are likely to find that their concentration and general thinking ability is much improved within weeks of starting a supplement containing pure EPA (without DHA) and virgin evening primrose oil. The Durham-Oxford trial that I mentioned in Chapter 5 showed a noticeable increase in reading age associated with just three months' fatty acid supplementation.

I know of the case of one child from a clinical study who had previously suffered from ADHD symptoms, being very restless, fidgety and unable to settle down and concentrate. Within just three months of taking an omega-3 and omega-6 fatty acid supplement, all these problems had disappeared. What was equally astonishing to his mother was that he suddenly started showing a strong interest in books. Rather than sitting in front of the television all evening, he now preferred to read. Before this particular study, I had thought that the malign influence of television was to blame for the general reduction in reading skills and reading for pleasure that we see in children (particularly boys) these days. I have had to revise my opinion in light of this and other examples. It now seems to me that perhaps children (and adults) find it easier and more enjoyable to read when they have higher levels of omega-3 and omega-6 fatty acids.

Cardiovascular system

Eskimo diet

In the 1950s, Dr Hugh Sinclair of Oxford University, mentor to Professor David Horrobin (who in turn was one of my mentors), discovered that the Inuit did not suffer from anywhere near as much heart disease and high blood pressure as those living in

Western countries, in spite of the fact that they ate large amounts of 'animal fats' such as fish and seals.

Clinically, one good way of looking at how furred up the arteries are is to look at the eyes. The coloured part of the eye, the iris, which surrounds the black pupil in the middle, gradually starts to develop an outer 'annular' whitish ring as hardening of the arteries and deposition of fat takes place in the arteries of the body. Surprisingly, Sinclair found that this annulus (known as an *arcus senilis*) did not seem to occur in the Inuit who were eating their traditional Eskimo diet, even when the individuals concerned were of advanced years. This finding furnished further evidence that the Eskimos' traditional diet is associated with a healthy cardiovascular system.

Although Hugh Sinclair attributed this healthy state of affairs to the Inuit's high dietary intake of omega-3 fatty acids, at first this explanation was rejected by some in the medical establishment. They argued instead that what Sinclair had discovered were the effects of a special genetic adaptation that had occurred during the many centuries that the Inuit population had spent genetically isolated from other human gene pools. In other words, this argument attributed the resistance of the Inuit to cardiovascular disease to their genes.

Evidence supporting Hugh Sinclair's contention came to light when epidemiological studies (studies of disease occurrence and behaviour across whole populations) were carried out on Inuit communities who had emigrated to Canada. When members of this population moved from their traditional high-omega-3 Eskimo diet to a Western diet, their levels of cardiovascular disease, including heart attacks and thrombotic strokes, rose to match that in the more indigenous Western populations around them. In fact, other diseases that had also appeared to be relatively uncommon in those Inuit on a high-omega-3 diet also rose to match those of people in the West generally once the Inuit changed their diets to a typical Western diet low in omega-3 fatty acids. These diseases included arthritis and other joint problems, diabetes and its complications such as neuropathy (nerve damage), and skin diseases such as eczema.

Benefits of high EPA

In addition to examining their eyes, Hugh Sinclair carried out another test that was fairly easy to perform in the Eskimo populations of Greenland without ready recourse to advanced laboratories and hospitals. This was to measure how quickly their blood clotted – in other words, how 'thin' their blood was .

Normally, if we cut ourselves, after a couple of minutes or so the cut stops bleeding as the previously oozing blood starts to clot and form a solid barrier. We need this to happen, but under certain circumstances, a propensity for blood to clot within a couple of minutes can be a distinct disadvantage. One such example is the tendency for blood clots to form in the blood vessels (deep veins) of the calf muscles of the lower leg following prolonged periods of inactivity, as may occur during a long-haul flight or even a long coach journey. This may cause tenderness of the calf and swelling of the lower leg. The individual may also start to suffer from a slight fever. On reaching his (or her) destination, the traveller will get up from his cramped sitting position and may dislodge the clot (or thrombus) or cause smaller clots to break off. In turn, these clots may then travel up his veins and, via the right-side of the heart, move into the major vessels in his lungs, where they may lodge. This is known as pulmonary embolism. Patients may become breathless, suffer from chest pain, find there is blood in their spit (sputum), become dizzy and faint. Their temperature and heart rate may rise, their blood pressure may fall, and they may develop bluish lips. If large clots lodge in the lungs, the patient may die. Since this condition starts with the formation of a clot or thrombus in deep veins, it is known as deep vein thrombosis, or DVT for short.

Quick blood clotting may have other disadvantages. For example, a clot may form in one of the coronary arteries that supply the heart with blood. This means that the part of the heart tissue that is deprived of a blood supply may start to die; this is a 'heart attack'. A final example relates to the occurrence of a clot in one of the blood vessels of the brain. If this happens, then the blood supply to part of the brain will be cut off, leading to damage and possible death of some brain tissue. This is a stroke (or, more accurately, a thrombotic stroke).

So, if your blood is 'thinner' and less likely to clot as a result of your taking a high dose of EPA, then there is clearly a reduced risk of suffering from deep vein thrombosis, or from pulmonary embolism, a heart attack or a thrombotic stroke.

If you have suffered from a deep-vein thrombosis, or from pulmonary embolism, a heart attack or a thrombotic stroke, then as part of your medical treatment you may be put on a blood thinning medicine. Initially this is often heparin, in the form of injections, while later, after discharge from hospital, it is likely to be warfarin, acenocoumarol or phenindione in the form of tablets. (Warfarin is also used as rat poison.) At the time of writing, a new blood thinning drug called ximelagastran (Exanta) has been approved for use in some parts of Europe. If you are on such medication, then you should consult your doctor if you decide to start taking a supplement of omega-3 fatty acids. This is so that the doctor can make any necessary adjustments to your blood thinning drugs, just in case your blood thins noticeably further as a result of taking the supplement. In practice, it is worth pointing out that a fatty acid supplement is unlikely to thin your blood to such an extent as to be noticeable. I have been taking eight VegEPA capsules daily for a long time, purely for the health benefits they give me, and all I have noticed are these benefits, without any bleeding problems at all; my blood does take longer to clot, which is a good thing, but I have not noticed any greater tendency to bruise.

Atrial fibrillation

The heart has four chambers, two upper 'atria' and two lower ventricles. In certain conditions, the upper atria, instead of pumping blood into the lower ventricles in a purposeful rhythmic manner, lose their rhythm and just seem to quiver, so that the heart is not as effective a pump as it should be. Conditions that can cause this condition, known as atrial fibrillation, include ischaemic heart disease (reduced blood supply to the muscles of the heart), problems with certain heart valves, rheumatic heart disease, high blood pressure, hyperthyroidism (thyrotoxicosis), heart surgery and pulmonary embolism.

Dr Dariush Mozaffarian, from Brigham and Women's Hospital and Harvard Medical School in Boston, Massachusetts, and colleagues, studied 4,815 adults aged 65 years or older in 1989 and 1990. Their assessments included details of their diet. During a 12-year follow-up period, in which the people studied had annual heart tracings (electrocardiograms) taken, there were 980 cases of atrial fibrillation. Analysis of the data showed that the higher their intake of tuna, or other broiled or baked fish, the lower their rate of atrial fibrillation. In other words, a high intake of omega-3 fatty acids appeared to be associated with a reduced risk of atrial fibrillation. These results were published in 2004 in the journal *Circulation*.

Joints

Arthritis afflicts increasing numbers of people as they get older. It is a condition in which there is inflammation of one or more of the joints in the body. The symptoms are pain, swelling, redness, stiffness and warmth of the joint or joints. The sufferer might also sometimes be feverish. A major form of arthritis is osteoarthritis, in which the protective cartilage around the ends of two bones that meet in the joint degenerates. The amount of the nourishing and cushioning fluid in the joint (known as synovial fluid) is also diminished as the osteoarthritis progresses. The resulting wearing action of one bone on the other, without sufficient intervening cartilage and synovial fluid, can cause excruciating pain.

Osteoarthritis and some cases of other types of arthritis (such as rheumatoid arthritis) can be helped by taking a combination of EPA and virgin evening primrose oil. The EPA helps restore the functioning of the synovial fluid in the joints, while a particularly important helpful component of virgin evening primrose oil is the family of triterpines that were described briefly in Chapter 6. (Triterpines help improve joint functioning by inhibiting certain enzymes.)

A suitable starting dose for adults with arthritis would be between four and eight VegEPA capsules daily, depending on the severity of the joint problems. For adolescents with juvenile arthritis, two to four capsules daily can be taken, depending on age.

Body weight

If an adult or child is not *underweight* to begin with, then they need not worry that taking a supplement such as VegEPA may cause an increase in their body weight. On the contrary, if anything, if you are overweight to begin with, you may well notice that you start to become slimmer once you are taking the supplement. If you are overweight, the supplement will make you feel full during a meal sooner than you are used to. So long as you stop eating when you do feel full, then you will gradually lose weight. (Obviously, if someone keeps eating even when they are not hungry, and takes little exercise, their calorie intake will exceed their calorie expenditure each day and they will inevitably put on weight – it is not possible to subvert the laws of physics.)

Skin, hair and nails

Within a few weeks of starting a fatty acid supplement containing pure EPA and virgin evening primrose oil, most people (whether or not they have been suffering from ADHD) begin to notice a striking improvement in their skin, hair and nails.

Those who have been suffering from dry skin notice that their skin is no longer dry but is being moisturized from the inside in a totally natural way. If they suffered from dry lips and/or a dry mouth, they find that these conditions also clear up, perhaps for the first time in many years. I have found that my patients' skin looks so much better that often their partners insist that they too want to start taking the supplement in order to benefit from the natural more youthful looking skin that it produces. There is absolutely no harm in doing this (so long as the person checks first with their doctor if they are taking a blood thinning drug such as warfarin or heparin). In fact, given the many benefits of EPA and virgin evening primrose oil, it could be argued that there is a case for actively encouraging people in general to take such a supplement. Regular supplementation with virgin evening primrose oil and EPA usually also helps clear up other skin conditions such as acne and eczema.

In addition to making your skin look much better and more youthful, omega-3 and omega-6 fatty acid supplements help keep hair glossy and better-looking. This is particularly noticeable if the individual previously suffered from dry hair, perhaps with split ends.

EPA combined with virgin evening primrose oil is also wonderfully good for your nails. Many people notice that, after the first three months, their nails are the best they can ever remember. Again, this is particularly noticeable if they were previously dry and brittle or unduly soft.

10
Treating ADHD Naturally

In this, the final chapter, I shall go through some practical issues related to the natural treatment of ADHD. First I shall describe how you can tell if you are deficient in omega-3 and omega-6 fatty acids. Next, I shall look at issues relating to omega-3 and omega-6 fatty acid supplementation, changes in diet, exercise and intellectual pursuits.

Fatty acid deficiency

Having carried out a thorough medical assessment, excluded the possibility of another illness and therefore confirmed the working clinical diagnosis of ADHD, the next thing I do in clinical practice is to assess the level of fatty acid deficiency. There are two ways of doing this. The method I prefer is to look for clinical features of fatty acid deficiency. The other way is to take a blood sample for measurement of the levels of omega-3 and omega-6 fatty acids in the membranes of the red blood cells.

Clinical features
There are several features that can be related to fatty acid deficiency. I have mentioned some of these earlier in the book. For convenience, I shall repeat them here. They include:

- Dry hair

- Problems with your nails – soft or brittle, for example

- Skin problems – dryness, roughness, eczema, psoriasis

- Suffering from dry lips for much of the day

- Suffering from a dry mouth for much of the day

- Usually feeling more thirsty than would be expected in the circumstances

- Poor sleep

- Having hands that become particularly cold or change colour sometimes, especially in winter

- Having feet that become particularly cold or change colour sometimes, especially in winter

- Needing to pass water more often than is usual for people of the same age

- Suffering from asthma, hayfever or other allergies.

Blood testing

Some specialized centres offer the facility to assess directly the level of omega-3 and omega-6 fatty acids in the membranes of your red blood cells. This is considered to be a good indicator of the state of the fatty acids in the membranes of organs such as the brain.

On page 176 I have listed typical normal reference ranges for some of the omega-3 and omega-6 fatty acids, for adults. This means that if the level measured is below the lower end of the range for that particular fatty acid, then you are deficient in that fatty acid. These figures are a guide only; in practice, if the laboratory you use offers a set of reference ranges, those should be used in preference to the ones listed here. Note that the figures are given as micromoles per litre. A mole, in this context, is a scientific measure referring to the mass (weight) of a substance that contains a certain specified number of molecules (or atoms) of that substance. For example, one mole of the commonest form of the element carbon, known as carbon-12, has a mass of exactly 12 grams. A micromole is one millionth of a mole. So a micromole of carbon-12 has a mass of 12 micrograms.

For the omega-6 fatty acids, typical normal reference ranges are:

- LA: 30 to 76 micromoles per litre

- GLA: 0.7 to 2.5 micromoles per litre

- DGLA: 5.0 to 9.7 micromoles per litre

- AA: 28 to 70 micromoles per litre.

For the omega-3 fatty acids, typical normal reference ranges are:

- ALA: 2.2 to 5.9 micromoles per litre

- EPA: 2.1 to 7.4 micromoles per litre.

Supplementation

For the reasons given in Chapter 7, the best omega-3 and omega-6 fatty acid supplement to take is one that contains a combination of pure EPA and virgin evening primrose oil (with preferably no DHA whatsoever). The one supplement currently available to the general public that fulfils these criteria is VegEPA. This can be obtained from the web site www.vegepa.com or from the telephone number or address given at the end of the book.

A good dose to start with for an adult with ADHD is eight of these capsules daily, taken for example as four each morning and four each evening, preferably with food. As mentioned earlier in the book, the dose for children aged between five and 12 years is two capsules daily, while for children aged between 12 and 16 years the dose is four capsules daily. The capsules are fairly small and easy to swallow. If swallowing is too difficult for any reason, then the capsules can be crunched in the mouth and the contents swallowed, though children may not like the taste. As mentioned before, it is even possible to cut open the vegetarian capsule shells and squeeze the contents into some fruit juice or yoghurt.

It can take at least three months for the full benefits to start to become apparent. Once improvement starts to occur, it is worth continuing with the treatment as the underlying problem with the enzyme delta-6-desaturase will not have gone away.

In the unlikely event that no benefits have been noticed at all after three months, it may be worth having the special test of fatty acids in the red blood cell membranes. This will show whether or not the EPA and omega-6 levels are in the normal range. If they are still rather low (particularly the EPA on the omega-3 side), in spite of taking the recommended daily dose, then there are several things you can do.

First, ensure that the ADHD sufferer is getting enough of the cofactors described in Chapter 8 (several B vitamins, vitamin C, zinc, selenium and magnesium). A good way of doing this is to ensure that their diet is adequate in these vitamins and trace elements; I have included further details of foods rich in these cofactors in that chapter. Another way of getting enough cofactors is to take vitamin and mineral supplements. The best way of obtaining these in supplement form is by taking either one mini-VegeCO tablet daily (for children between the ages of 6 and 12 years), or two mini-VegeCO tablets daily (for children aged over 12 years). Adults should take one VegeCO tablet daily.

Second, the ADHD sufferer may be under too much stress in their daily life. For children this may result from bullying or excessive academic pressure, perhaps made all the worse by comorbid dyslexia or developmental coordination disorder. For adults, the stress could be caused by work colleagues, financial problems, relationship difficulties, concern about relatives, or a host of other reasons. Unfortunately, long-running raised stress levels can in turn raise the levels of stress hormones such as cortisol, which in turn inhibit the proper functioning of the enzyme delta-6-desaturase. This enzyme is involved in the conversion of

EPA into natural DHA, and so it is good to try to reduce the levels of stress. Good stress-busters include exercise and certain complementary therapies (see below), as well as altering the way people think about the things that make them feel stressed. If it comes to the worst, it may be worth making some major lifestyle changes to make life less stressful.

The third thing that can be done is temporarily to raise the intake of the supplement, by an extra capsule each day. After three months, the dose can be brought back down to the recommended amounts given above.

Caffeine, alcohol and smoking

It is possible that caffeine, alcohol and nicotine may inhibit the action of the enzyme delta-6-desaturase. If possible, ADHD sufferers should therefore try to reduce their intake of caffeine-containing drinks, such as coffee, cola drinks and tea. If you are an adult ADHD sufferer and drink heavily, it would be better to reduce your alcohol consumption to only a moderate amount.

As for nicotine, there is no question that it is extremely bad for your health to smoke. If you are a smoker, you should make every effort to give up. Nowadays there are many aids to stopping smoking. If you need help, ask your family doctor.

Diet

Cofactors
As I described in Chapter 8, it is important to eat a healthy diet that is rich in the following cofactors:

- Folic acid

- Vitamin B_{12}

- Vitamin B_6

- Niacin

- Biotin

- Vitamin C

- Zinc

- Selenium, and

- Magnesium.

You should go through each of these cofactors in turn, and check that you (or your child) are regularly eating at least one of the foodstuffs that are a good source of each one. (The relevant lists are given in Chapter 8.)

Manufactured trans fats

When making margarine, vegetable oils are industrially changed to turn them into solids at room temperature. This process is known as hydrogenation, and the result is hydrogenated vegetable fat. Unfortunately, the industrial processes involved cause the fatty acids in the vegetable oil to be turned into strange molecules called trans fats. (The trans in this name refers to a special type of chemical bond in the molecules called trans bonds.)

When ingested, the body treats the trans fats as if they were ordinary naturally occurring fatty acids. This causes at least two sets of profound problems for our health.

First, trans fats inhibit the action of the enzyme delta-6-desaturase. As explained below in the section on cortisol, this means that it becomes more difficult for the body to produce DHA (from EPA). In addition, it also means it is more difficult for the body to produce EPA, DGLA and AA from the dietary fatty acid precursors; this should not be a problem, though, if you (or your child) are taking a supplement containing pure EPA and virgin evening primrose oil, as you (or your child) can then produce your own DGLA and AA from the virgin evening primrose oil.

The second problem is that the cells of our bodies, including those of the brain, unfortunately incorporate the trans fats into their membranes. This makes the membranes very inflexible. In turn, membrane receptors do not work properly and signals do not pass properly between cells. This includes problems with signals passing between brain cells.

The best policy is to remove trans fats from the diet and to put the ADHD sufferer on a high pure EPA and virgin evening primrose oil supplement. But which 'foods' contain these artificial trans fats? Unfortunately, the answer is very many processed foodstuffs that contain hydrogenated fat, including:

- Margarine

- Pastries

- Bread (if the ingredients include 'hydrogenated vegetable oil')

- Most biscuits (unless made with pure butter)

- Most cakes (unless made with pure butter)

- Most pies

- Pre-packed sachets of drinking chocolate and of some coffee preparations.

If you look carefully at the ingredients list on the products you buy, you should be able to avoid most sources.

Butter is an excellent alternative to margarine. It is particularly good to go for a brand of butter that is derived from cows that never eat concentrated feedstock or get confined to sheds. An excellent brand that is widely available is Anchor Butter, from New Zealand. The cows for Anchor Butter roam free and eat fresh green grass all year round. As a result, this particular brand of butter should also contain some EPA (unlike butter from grain-fed cows).

Fried foods

Frying is generally bad for you, as the high temperatures involved harm the omega-3 fatty acids in foods such as fish, as well as producing artificial poisons such as acrylamide. In the study by Dr Dariush Mozaffarian and colleagues, published in 2004 and described in the previous chapter, there was a very interesting finding: while a diet rich in fish containing omega-3 fatty acids was found to reduce the risk of atrial fibrillation, this protective effect of dietary fish did not apply to fish that had been fried.

Suitable alternatives to frying are steaming or lightly grilling your food. You are less likely to create acrylamide by steaming your food, and both steaming and light grilling are less likely than frying to harm the omega-3 fatty acids in your food. (Acrylamide is a potential carcinogen that is formed when carbohydrate-rich foods are fried, baked, grilled, toasted or microwaved at temperatures above 120 degrees Celsius.)

Sugar

Ordinary sugar (or sucrose), particularly white sugar, can harm your body in many ways. One of these relates to its effects on energy levels. After the immediate rush that occurs following a meal or drink that contains added sugar, your energy levels may actually feel as if they have diminished, as your body tries hard to mop up all the extra sugar by pouring out insulin into your bloodstream. In order to cope with the feeling of tiredness that this process engenders, you may have another sugar-containing 'food' or drink. And so the cycle repeats itself day after day through endless cups of sweet tea and coffee, and large numbers of chocolate bars, sweets and biscuits (laden with harmful trans fats). Eventually, your body may no longer be able to cope and diabetes mellitus will start to develop.

Excessive consumption of sugar-sweetened soft drinks may also be contributing to the relentless rise in childhood obesity in many countries.

If you (or your child) feel peckish in between your three main meals of the day (and I do strongly recommend that you do try to have three square meals daily), then try some of the following possibilities:

- Fresh fruit – bananas, apples, satsumas, pears, strawberries, blackcurrants, peaches, melons, among others, are all nutritious and can involve next-to-no preparation time

- Dried fruits – dates, figs and currants are particularly good ways of obtaining extra energy and also contain many valuable minerals

- Freshly squeezed orange juice or freshly pressed apple or pineapple juice – you should avoid 'fruit juices' made from concentrates, and, of course, always avoid 'fruit drinks' that contain added sugar

- A glass of whole milk, with a honey sandwich (made with wholemeal bread and butter)

- A carton of natural yoghurt perhaps sweetened with some honey.

In the next section, I shall give you the ingredients of a good breakfast.

Cortisol

As I described earlier in this book, high levels of the hormone cortisol circulating in the blood can inhibit the action of the enzyme delta-6-desaturase. This enzyme occurs twice in Figure 13 (see page 81). First, it is used to help convert the parent, or precursor, short-chain essential fatty acids LA and ALA into their respective omega-6 and omega-3 fatty acid long-chain derivatives. Second, delta-6-desaturase is one of the enzymes that helps in the conversion of EPA into DHA. For the reasons explained in Chapter 7, you should avoid taking any DHA in supplements. This means that the DHA you need should be derived from EPA within your body, using your (limited, if you have ADHD) supply of delta-6-desaturase. To give the enzyme as much help as possible it is therefore important to reduce the circulating levels of cortisol.

Levels of the steroid hormone cortisol rise in the blood as a result of stresses such as:

- Anxiety

- Fear

- Pain

- Infections

- Low blood sugar levels

- Haemorrhage (bleeding), and

- Starvation.

So, to reduce the circulating cortisol levels, you should work on trying to reduce these factors in your (or your child's) life.

Try to learn to cope with circumstances that make you anxious or fearful. Exercise, and some of the complementary therapies mentioned below, should help here. You could also ask your doctor to refer you for cognitive behavioural therapy, or CBT for short, which is a short form of psychotherapy that some patients find helpful. (In cognitive behavioural therapy, the therapist helps correct negative thought patterns and low self-image from which the patient may suffer.)

You should certainly avoid pain. You should also try to ensure that you (and your children) do not go without three well-balanced proper meals daily, so that your blood sugar levels do not drop during the day. Make time for a good nourishing breakfast each day. My usual breakfast, which helps set me up for the long working day ahead consists of:

- Muesli (made without added sugar or salt) that is rich in dried fruits, nuts and seeds

- Honey to sweeten the muesli

- Full-cream whole fresh milk – sometimes I prepare the muesli the evening before by adding milk to a bowl of it and leaving it in the refrigerator overnight

- A glass of freshly squeezed orange juice

- Four VegEPA capsules – I take my other four capsules each evening.

Avoid allowing your body weight to become so low that your body interprets this as starvation and raises the levels of cortisol.

Exercise

Most children with ADHD do not have to be asked twice to take the opportunity to engage in physical exercise. The problem for many of them is limited opportunity to take exercise in a constructive way as the time for PE (physical exercise/education) in schools has been greatly reduced and modern life is increasingly restrictive for many children as their parents struggle to keep them safe from traffic, 'stranger danger', and worse. As I mentioned before, parents of ADHD children often find themselves being particularly restrictive because their children have very little sense of danger. Organizing after-school physical activities like football or swimming should help, though this can be stressful in their own right if there is too much emphasis on good behaviour and motor coordination.

For adult ADHD sufferers, gentle exercise is an excellent stress-buster; good forms of exercise include:

- Walking – particularly enjoyable if you have a friend or partner to accompany you

- Cycling, and

- Swimming.

Complementary therapies

There are several types of complementary therapy that can help relax the muscles and act as stress-busters.

Massage therapy
For adult sufferers there are various forms of massage therapy available. They are good ways of helping you to feel more relaxed and less stressed. In one form, Shiatsu, the practitioner will carry out a form of acupressure in which certain points in the body are especially stimulated, perhaps by the use of the thumbs, fingers, elbows or even knees.

Aromatherapy
Aromatherapy involves massaging essential oils into the skin. Your aromatherapist will be able to choose the most appropriate essential oils for your particular symptoms. In addition, you might want to consider using essential oils to help you or your child relax or sleep. For example, you could try putting one or two drops of lavender oil on the pillow case when going to bed. Inhaling the vapour from this oil might help you or your child to sleep better.

The Alexander Technique
If you can find a good teacher, then the Alexander Technique has much to commend it. It is a method of mind and body re-education that can help to reduce stress and muscular tension. It also acts at a deep, unconscious level, to enable personal growth to take place. Some practitioners are willing to take on pupils under the age of 16 years. A good introduction can be found in the books *The Alexander Principle: How to Use Your Body without Stress* by Dr Wilfred Barlow and *Body Learning: An Introduction to the Alexander Technique* by Michael Gelb.

Intellectual pursuits

As an ADHD child recovers on fatty acid supplementation, it is important to provide them with an intellectually enriching environment. Take them to your local public library at least twice every week. Organize visits to museums. Take them to public talks, music concerts and the theatre. Surround them with books and encourage them to become avid readers. Above all, do not let them waste their life away becoming television addicts. As their attention and concentration improve on the fatty acids, encourage them to read rather than watch television programmes or play computer games.

Conclusion

As I said at the start of this book, the result of a recent major research breakthrough means that there is now, at long last, excellent news for people whose lives are devastated by ADHD. This breakthrough is in our understanding of fatty acids, how their absence can cause the symptoms of ADHD, and how they can safely be used to treat sufferers from this condition, children and adults alike.

Glossary

AA: arachidonic acid – a long chain polyunsaturated fatty omega-6 fatty acid created from GLA via DGLA or eaten in the diet. It is of vital importance as a building block for eicosanoids.

Adrenal glands: glands lying just above the kidneys. The outer part of the glands secrete the stress hormone cortisol. The adrenal glands are sometimes also called the suprarenal glands.

Adrenic acid: an omega-6 long-chain polyunsaturated fatty acid. It is formed from arachidonic acid.

ALA: alpha-linolenic acid – the essential (short chain) parent omega-3 fatty acid.

Alpha-linolenic acid: the essential (short chain) parent omega-3 fatty acid.

Amino acid: a building block of proteins.

Amphetamine: a powerful psychostimulant. It is used to treat ADHD. It is a drug of addiction in adults.

Antibodies: special chemicals released by certain white blood cells (B lymphocytes). They bind to pathogenic organisms and their products. This allows pathogens to be identified by other white blood cells (phagocytes) which can then 'go in for the kill'.

Anticoagulant therapy: treatment (such as heparin, warfarin, acenocoumarol or phenindione) used to thin the blood.

Arachidonic acid: a long chain polyunsaturated omega-6 fatty acid created from the GLA via DGLA or eaten in the diet. It is of vital importance as a building block for eicosanoids.

Cardiomyopathy: a pathological condition in which the heart is enlarged.

Choline: a molecule that forms a polar head group in phospholipids.

Choreiform movements: involuntary abnormal, rapid, complex, jerky movements.

Clumsy child syndrome: another term for dyspraxia (see below).

Cofactors: certain vitamins and minerals that are needed to help the body properly utilize fatty acids.

Comorbidity: the co-occurrence of certain disorders. For example, ADHD often occurs with dyslexia and/or dyspraxia.

Cortisol: a steroid hormone produced by the outer part of the adrenal glands (the adrenal cortex). Its levels rise in the blood as a result of stresses such as anxiety, fear, pain, infections, low blood sugar levels, haemorrhage and starvation. It inhibits the enzyme delta-6-desaturase.

DEA: the United States Drug Enforcement Administration.

Delta-6-desaturase: an enzyme that has two important functions in the synthesis of fatty acids. First, it is used to help convert the parent essential fatty acids, linoleic acid and alpha-linolenic acid, into their respective omega-6 and omega-3 fatty acid derivatives, respectively. Second, delta-6-desaturase is one of the enzymes that helps in the conversion of EPA into DHA.

Deoxyribonucleic acid: also known as DNA. This is the main molecule of heredity, which carries genetic information through the generations.

Developmental coordination disorder: the DSM-IV-TR term for dyspraxia.

DGLA: dihomo-gamma-linolenic acid – an omega-6 long chain polyunsaturated fatty acid that the body can convert into arachidonic acid. It is of vital importance as a building block for eicosanoids.

DHA: docosahexaenoic acid – an omega-3 long chain polyunsaturated fatty acid that can be made from EPA. It is important in maintaining the correct structure of cell membranes.

Dihomo-gamma-linolenic acid: an omega-6 long chain polyunsaturated fatty acid that the body can convert into arachidonic acid. It is of vital importance as a building block for eicosanoids.

DNA: Deoxyribonucleic acid - the main molecule of heredity, which carries genetic information through the generations.

Docosahexaenoic acid: an omega-3 long chain polyunsaturated fatty acid that can be made from EPA. It is important in maintaining the correct structure of cell membranes.

Double-blind clinical trial: a research study involving both an active putative treatment and a placebo in which both the patients and the doctors or researchers do not know who is taking the active treatment and who the placebo during the whole course of the actual trial.

DSM-IV-TR: *The Diagnostic and Statistical Manual of Mental Disorders*, fourth edition, Text Revision published by the American Psychiatric Association.

Dyslexia: Literally, 'difficulty with words'. Language is processed abnormally, so that there is difficulty in skills such as reading, writing and spelling.

Dyspraxia: Difficulty with or impairment of the organization of movement.

Eicosanoids: families of thromboxanes, prostaglandins, leukotrienes and hydroxy fatty acids. These are of importance in maintaining the health of cells and tissues.

Eicosapentaenoic acid: an omega-3 long chain polyunsaturated fatty acid that is of vital importance as a building block for eicosanoids, sleep mediators, and interferons. It is viricidal (kills viruses).

Enzyme: a biological catalyst that helps chemical reactions to take place much faster.

EPA: eicosapentaenoic acid – an omega-3 long chain polyunsaturated fatty acid that is of vital importance as a building block for eicosanoids, sleep mediators, and interferons. It is viricidal (kills viruses).

Endocrine system: a system consisting of a number of hormone-secreting organs such as the pancreas and adrenal glands.

Essential fatty acids: the parent omega-3 and omega-6 fatty acids linoleic acid and alpha-linolenic acid.

Ethyl-EPA: an ethyl ester form of EPA that is ultra-pure. It is the form of EPA that has been used in many major research studies and is the form that biotechnology companies are trying to bring to the market for the treatment of illnesses such as depression, Huntington's disease and schizophrenia. It is also the form of pure EPA that is found in VegEPA.

Evening primrose oil: oil from the seeds of the evening primrose plant. It is rich in the omega-6 fatty acid GLA.

Gamma-linoleic acid: an omega-6 long chain polyunsaturated fatty acid that the body can convert into DGLA.

GLA: gamma-linoleic acid – an omega-6 long chain polyunsaturated fatty acid that the body can convert into DGLA.

Highly unsaturated fatty acid: an unsaturated fatty acid containing several double bonds between carbon atoms. Examples are EPA and GLA.

Hormones: chemical substances produced by endocrine and other glands. They circulate in the blood and influence various bodily functions.

HUFA: a commonly used abbreviation for highly unsaturated fatty acid.

Hydrogenated fats: these are the result of artificial processes in which vegetable oils, which are liquid at room temperature, are turned into hardened solids that are rich in trans fats.

Hyperkinetic disorders: According to the ICD-10, this is a group of disorders characterized by: early onset; a combination of over active, poorly modulated behaviour with marked inattention and lack of persistent task involvement; and pervasiveness over situations and persistence over time of these behavioural characteristics. Hyperkinetic disorder is a severe form of ADHD.

ICD-10: The *International Classification of Diseases* published by the World Health Organization.

LA: linoleic acid - the essential (short-chain) parent omega-6 fatty acid.

Linoleic acid: the essential (short chain) parent omega-6 fatty acid.

Methylphenidate: An artificial psychostimulant that is widely used for the treatment of ADHD.

Micromole: A micromole is one millionth of a mole. So a micromole of carbon-12 has a mass of 12 micrograms.

Microgram: A unit of mass (weight). A microgram is one-millionth of a gram, and one-billionth of a kilogram.

Milligram: A unit of mass (weight). A milligram is one-thousandth of a gram, and one millionth of a kilogram. The scientific abbreviation for milligram is mg.

Mole: A mole is a scientific measure referring to the mass (weight) of a substance that contains a certain specified number of molecules (or atoms) of that substance. For example, one mole of the commonest form of the element carbon, known as carbon-12, has a mass of exactly 12 grams. The scientific abbreviation for mole is mol.

Neurotransmitter: a chemical such as dopamine or serotonin that jumps across the gap between nerve cells, thereby allowing messages to pass from one nerve cell to another.

Niacin: a B vitamin.

Omega-3 fatty acids: a family of fatty acids that includes ALA, EPA and DHA.

Omega-6 fatty acids: a family of fatty acids that includes LA, GLA, DGLA and AA.

Organic driveness: An historical term, dating from the 1930s, in which it was suggested that the hyperactivity syndrome was caused by an organic disorder affecting the brain stem.

Phospholipid: a complex molecule found in all cell membranes that include fatty acids.

Placebo: an inactive or 'dummy' substance that looks identical to the active treatment in a double-blind trial.

Polyunsaturated fatty acid: an unsaturated fatty acid containing at least one double bond between carbon atoms. Examples are EPA and GLA.

Prostaglandins: important families of substances formed from fatty acids such as EPA that are essential for the well-being of the body.

Psychostimulant: A drug such as amphetamine or cocaine that strongly stimulates the brain.

PUFA: a commonly used abbreviation for polyunsaturated fatty acid.

Ritalin: A trade name for methylphenidate.

Thromboxanes: special derivatives of fatty acids that are needed for the well-being of the body.

Tics: Involuntary repetitive movements or, in the case of vocal tics, involuntary repetitive grunts or verbal utterances (sometimes of an offensive nature).

Trace elements: mineral elements that are needed in the diet in trace amounts.

Trans fats: the artificial trans fats are created in the industrial process of manufacturing hydrogenated fats. They have deleterious effects on cell membranes.

Trans fatty acids: another name for trans fats.

Triterpines: naturally occurring molecules that have several health-giving properties. They are found in virgin evening primrose oil.

Ventricles: chambers in the brain or heart, each of which has two ventricles.

Virgin evening primrose oil: evening primrose oil that is cold-pressed and non-raffinated so that it retains much of its goodness, including the presence of triterpines.

Working memory: The temporary storage of information in connection with performing other, more complex, tasks.

References

Aman, M.G., Mitchell, E.A. and Turbott, S.H. (1987). The effects of essential fatty acid supplementation by Efamol in hyperactive children. *Journal of Abnormal Child Psychology* **15**: 75-90.

American Heart Association (2002). AHA Scientific Statement: Fish Consumption, Fish Oil, Omega-3 Fatty Acids and Cardiovascular Disease, #71-0241. *Circulation* **106**: 2747-2757.

American Psychiatric Association (2000). *Diagnostic and Statistical Manual of Mental Disorders, 4th edition, Text Revision (DSM-IV-TR)*. American Psychiatric Association: Washington, D.C.

Arnold, L.E., Kleykamp, D., Votolato, N.A., Taylor, W.A., Kontras, S.B. and Tobin, K. (1989). Gamma-linolenic acid for attention-deficit hyperactivity disorder: placebo-controlled comparison to D-amphetamine. *Biological Psychiatry* **25**: 222-228.

Auster, S. (1999). Attention deficit disorder. *Pediatrics* **104**: 1419-1420.

Baddeley, A.D. and Hitch, G. (1974). Working memory. In: Bower, G.A. (editor) *The Psychology of Learning and Motivation*, volume 8. Academic Press: New York.

Barlow, W. (2001). *The Alexander Principle: How to Use Your Body without Stress*. London: Orion.

Bekaroglu, M., Aslan, Y., Gedik, Y., Deger, O., Mocan, H., Erduran, E. and Karahan, C. (1996). Relationships between serum free fatty acids and zinc, and attention deficit hyperactivity disorder: a research note. *Journal of Child Psychology and Psychiatry* **37**: 225-227.

Biederman, J., Wilens, T.E., Mick, E., Faraone, S.V. and Spencer, T. (1998). Does attention-deficit hyperactivity disorder impact the developmental course of drug and alcohol abuse and dependence? *Biological Psychiatry* **44**: 269-273.

Blum, K., Sheridan, P.J., Wood, R.C., Braverman, E.R., Chen, T.J., Cull, J.G. and Comings, D.E. (1996). The D2 dopamine receptor gene as a determinant of reward deficiency syndrome. *Journal of the Royal Society of Medicine* **89**: 396-400.

Bourre, J.M., Francois, M., Youyou, A., Dumont, O., Piciotti, M., Pascal, G. and Durand, G. (1989). The effects of dietary alpha-linolenic acid on the composition of nerve membranes, enzymatic activity, amplitude of electrophysiological parameters, resistance to poisons and performance of learning tasks in rats. *Journal of Nutrition* **119**: 1880-1892.

Bradley, C. (1937). The behavior of children receiving Benzedrine. *American Journal of Psychiatry* **94**: 577-585.

Buitelaar, J.K. (2002). Epidemiology of attention-deficit/hyperactivity disorder: what have we learned over the last decade? In: Sandberg, S. (editor) *Hyperactivity Disorders*. Cambridge University Press: Cambridge, pp. 30-63.

Chen, J.R., Hsu, S.F., Hsu, C.D., Hwang, L.H. and Yang, S.C. (2004). Dietary patterns and blood fatty acid composition in children with attention-deficit hyperactivity disorder in Taiwan. *Journal of Nutritional Biochemistry* **15**: 467-472.

Conners, C.K. (1997). *Conners' Parent Rating Scales - Revised*. Multi Health Systems Inc.: New York.

Conners, C.K. (1997). *Conners' Teacher Rating Scales - Revised: Long Form*. Multi Health Systems Inc.: New York.

Cornish, K.M., Manly, T., Savage, R., Swanson, J., Morisano, D.,

Butler, N., Grant, C., Cross, G., Bentley, L. and Hollis, C.P. (2005). Association of the dopamine transporter (DAT1) 10/10-repeat genotype with ADHD symptoms and response inhibition in a general population sample. *Molecular Psychiatry* (in press).

Crawford, M.A. (1992). Essential fatty acids and neurodevelopmental disorder. In: Bazan, N.G. (editor) *Neurobiology of Essential Fatty Acids*. Plenum Press: New York, pp. 307-314.

Dale, R.C., Church, A.J., Surtees, R.A., Lees, A.J., Adcock, J.E., Harding, B., Neville, B.G. and Giovannoni, G. (2004). Encephalitis lethargica syndrome: 20 new cases and evidence of basal ganglia autoimmunity. *Brain* 127: 21-33.

Dandy, W.E. (1918). Ventriculography following the injection of air into the cerebral ventricles. *Annals of Surgery, Philadelphia* **68**: 5-11.

Dandy, W.E. (1919). Röntgenography of the brain after the injection of air into the spinal canal. *Annals of Surgery, Philadelphia* **70**: 397-403.

Darwin, C. (1859). *On the Origin of Species by Means of Natural Selection, or the Preservation of Favoured Races in the Struggle for Life*. John Murray: London, England.

De Vriese, S.R., Christophe, A.B. and Maes, M. (2004). In humans, the seasonal variation in poly-unsaturated fatty acids is related to the seasonal variation in violent suicide and serotonergic markers of violent suicide. *Prostaglandins Leukotrienes and Essential Fatty Acids* **71**: 13-18.

Delion, S., Chalon, S., Guilloteau, D., Besnard, J.C. and Durand, G. (1996). ±-Linolenic acid dietary deficiency alters age-related changes of dopaminergic and serotoninergic neurotransmission in the rat frontal cortex.*Journal of Neurochemistry* **66**: 1582-1591.

Delion, S., Chalon, S., Herault, J., Guilloteau, D., Besnard, J.C. and Durand, G. (1994). Chronic dietary ±-linolenic acid deficiency alters dopaminergic and serotoninergic neurotransmission in rats. *Journal of Nutrition* **124**: 2466-2476.

Dobler, V.B., Anker, S., Gilmore, J., Robertson, I.H., Atkinson, J. and Manly, T. (2005). Asymmetric deterioration of spatial awareness with diminishing levels of alertness in normal children and children with ADHD. *Journal of Child Psychology and Psychiatry* (in press).

Durston, S., Fossella, J.A., Casey, B.J., Hulshoff Pol, H.E., Galvan, A., Schnack, H.G., Steenhuis, M.P., Minderaa, R.B., Buitelaar, J.K., Kahn, R.S. and van Engeland, H. (2005). Differential effects of DRD4 and DAT1 genotype on fronto-striatal gray matter volumes in a sample of subjects with attention deficit hyperactivity disorder, their unaffected siblings, and controls. *Molecular Psychiatry* (in press).

Erubin 54b (1938). In: Epstein, I. (editor); Slotki, I.W. (translator) *The Babylonian Talmud; Seder Mo'ed, Volume 2.* The Soncino Press: London, England p. 383.

Fagioli, I., Baroncini, P., Ricour, C. and Salzarulo, P. (1989). Decrease of slow-wave sleep in children with prolonged absence of essential lipids intake. *Sleep* **12**: 495-499.

Gelb, M.J. (2004). *Body Learning: An Introduction to the Alexander Technique.* London: Aurum Press.

Gillberg, C., Rasmussen, P., Carlstrom, G., Svenson, B. and Waldenstrom, E. (1982). Perceptual, motor and attentional deficits in six-year-old children. Epidemiological aspects. *Journal of Child Psychology and Psychiatry* **23**: 131-144.

Graham, J. (1984). *Evening Primrose Oil: Its Remarkable Properties and its Use in the Treatment of a Wide Range of Conditions.* Wellingborough, Northamptonshire, U.K.: Thorsons Publishers Ltd.

Hagberg, B. (1975). Vad innebär det för barnets utveckling och anpassning. [Minimal brain dysfunction.] *Läkartidningen* **72**: 3296-3300.

Hall, C. (2005). Children's drug can cause liver damage. *Daily Telegraph* 4 Feb.

Hamburger, M., Riese, U., Graf, H., Melzig, M.F., Ciesielski, S., Baumann, D., Dittmann, K. and Wegner, C. (2002). Constituents in evening primrose oil with radical scavenging, cyclooxygenase, and neutrophil elastase inhibitory activities. *Journal of Agricultural and Food Chemistry* **50**: 5533-5538

Harding, K.L., Judah, R.D. and Gant, C.E. (2003). Outcome-based comparison of Ritalin® versus food-supplement treated children with AD/HD. *Alternative Medicine Review* **8**: 319-330.

Hibbeln, J.R. (1998). Fish consumption and major depression. *Lancet* **351**: 1213.

Hirayama, S., Hamazaki, T. and Terasawa, K. (2004). Effect of docosahexaenoic acid-containing food administration on symptoms of attention-deficit/hyperactivity disorder - a placebo-controlled double-blind study. *European Journal of Clinical Nutrition* **58**: 467-473.

Hoffmann, H. (1846). *Der Struwwelpeter: oder Lustige Geschichten und Drollige Bilder für Kinder von 3-6 Jahren.* (Second edition.) English edition: *Slovenly Peter or Cheerful Stories and Funny Pictures for Good Little Folks.* John C. Winston: Philadelphia, PA, USA.

Kahn, E. and Cohen, L.H. (1934). Organic driveness: A brain stem syndrome and an experience. *New England Journal of Medicine* **210**: 748-756.

Kanner, L. (1957). *Child Psychiatry, third edition.* Blackwell Scientific: Oxford, England.

Laking, P.J. (2003). Child and Adolescent Psychiatry. In: Puri, B.K., Laking, P.J. and Treasaden, I.H. *Textbook of Psychiatry, 2nd edition.* Churchill Livingstone: Edinburgh, pp. 317-345.

Leung, P.W., Lee, C.C., Hung, S.F., Ho, T.P., Tang, C.P., Kwong, S.L., Leung, S.Y., Yuen, S.T., Lieh-Mak, F., Oosterlann, J., Grady., D., Harxhi, A., Ding., Y.C., Chi, H.C., Flodman, P., Schuck, S., Spence., M.A., Moyzis, R. and Swanson, J. (2005). Dopamine receptor D4 (DRD4) gene in Han Chinese children with attention-deficit/hyperactivity disorder (ADHD): increased prevalence of the 2-repeat allele. *American Journal of Medical Genetics Part B: Neuropsychiatric Genetics* **133**: 54-56.

Maes, M., Cosyns, P., Meltzer, H.Y., De Meyer, F. and Peeters, D. (1993). Seasonality in violent suicide but not in nonviolent suicide or homicide. *American Journal of Psychiatry* **150**: 1380-1385.

Maes, M., Meltzer, H.Y., Suy, E. and De Meyer, F. (1993). Seasonality in severity of depression: relationships to suicide and homicide occurrence. *Acta Psychiatrica Scandinavica* **88**: 156-161.

Martino, D. and Giovannoni, G. (2004). Antibasal ganglia antibodies and their relevance to movement disorders. *Current Opinion in Neurology* **17**: 425-432.

Mitchell, E.A., Aman, M.G., Turbott, S.H. and Manku, M. (1987). Clinical characteristics and serum essential fatty acid levels in hyperactive children. *Clinical Pediatrics* **26**: 406-411.

Mozaffarian, D., Psaty, B.M., Rimm, E.B., Lemaitre, R.N., Burke, G.L., Lyles, M.F., Lefkowitz, D. and Siscovick, D.S. (2004). Fish intake and risk of incident atrial fibrillation. *Circulation* **110**: 368-373.

National Institute for Clinical Excellence (NICE) (2000). *Technology Appraisal Guidance - Number 13. Guidance on the Use of Methylphenidate (Ritalin, Equasym) for Attention Deficit/ Hyperactivity Disorder (ADHD) in Childhood.* October 2000.

Nemets, B., Stahl, Z. and Belmaker, R.H. (2002). Addition of Omega-3 Fatty Acid to Maintenance Medication Treatment for Recurrent Unipolar Depressive Disorder. *American Journal of Psychiatry* **159**: 477-479.

Neuringer, M., Anderson, G.J. and Connor, W.E. (1988). The essentiality of n-3 fatty acids for the development and function of the retina and brain. *Annual Review of Nutrition* **8**: 517-541.

Olds, J. and Milner, P. (1954). Positive reinforcement produced by electrical stimulation of septal area and other regions of rat brain. *Journal of Comparative and Physiological Psychology* **47**: 419-427.

Pauling, L. (1972) *Vitamin C and the Common Cold.* London: Ballantine Books.

Peet, M. and Horrobin, D.F. (2002). A dose-ranging study of the effects of ethyl-eicosapentaenoate in patients with ongoing depression despite apparently adequate treatment with standard drugs. *Archives of General Psychiatry* **59**: 913-919.

Pomerleau, O.F., Downey, K.K., Stelson, F.W. and Pomerleau, C.S. (1995). Cigarette smoking in adult patients diagnosed with attention deficit hyperactivity disorder. *Journal of Substance Abuse* **7**: 373-378.

Portwood, M. (1999). *Developmental Dyspraxia: Identification and Intervention: A Manual for Parents and Professionals*. David Fulton: London, England.

Portwood, M., Lowerson, S.A. and Puri, B.K. (2005). High-eicosapentaenoic acid-containing long-chain polyunsaturated fatty acid supplementation in drug-naïve children with developmental coordination disorder and childhood-occurring dyslexia and attention-deficit hyperactivity disorder symptomatology: a randomised double-blind placebo-controlled clinical trial. *Prostaglandins, Leukotrienes and Essential Fatty Acids* (in press).

Puri, B.K. (2004). The clinical advantages of cold-pressed non-raffinated evening primrose oil over refined preparations. *Medical Hypotheses* **62**: 116-118.

Puri, B.K. (2005). *Chronic Fatigue Syndrome*. Hammersmith Press: London.

Puri, B.K. and Boyd, H. (2004). *The Natural Way to Beat Depression: The Groundbreaking Discovery of EPA to Change Your Life*. Hodder Mobius: London.

Puri, B.K. and Richardson, A.J. (2000). The effects of olive oil on omega-3 fatty acids and mood disorder. *Archives of General Psychiatry* **57**: 715.

Puri, B.K., Counsell, S.J., Hamilton, G., Richardson, A.J. and Horrobin, D.F. (2001). Eicosapentaenoic acid in treatment-resistant depression associated with symptom remission, structural brain changes and reduced neuronal phospholipid turnover. *International Journal of Clinical Practice* **55**: 560-563.

Puri, B.K., Counsell, S.J., Richardson, A.J. and Horrobin, D.F. (2002). Eicosapentaenoic acid in treatment-resistant depression. *Archives of General Psychiatry* **59**: 91-92.

Puri, B.K., El-Dosoky, A. and Barrett, J.S. (1994). Self-inflicted intracranial injury. *British Journal of Psychiatry* **164**: 841-842.

Puri, B.K., Laking, P.J. and Treasaden, I.H. (2002). *Textbook of Psychiatry, 2nd edition.* Churchill Livingstone: Edinburgh.

Quinn, P. and Wigal, S. (2004). Perceptions of girls and ADHD: results from a national survey. *Medscape General Medicine* **6(2)**.

Richardson, A.J. (2003). Clinical trials of fatty acid supplementation in dyslexia and dyspraxia, in *Phospholipid Spectrum Disorder in Psychiatry and Neurology, 2nd edn.* (Peet, M., Glen, I. and Horrobin, D.F., eds.), Marius Press, Carnforth, Lancashire, pp. 491-500.

Richardson, A.J. and Montgomery, P. (2005). The Oxford-Durham study: a randomized, controlled trial of dietary supplementation with fatty acids in children with developmental coordination disorder. *Pediatrics* **115**: 1360-1366.

Richardson, A.J. and Puri, B.K. (2000). The potential role of fatty acids in attention-deficit/hyperactivity disorder. *Prostaglandins Leukotrienes and Essential Fatty Acids* **63**: 79-87.

Richardson, A.J. and Puri, B.K. (2002). A randomized double-blind, placebo-controlled study of the effects of supplementation with highly unsaturated fatty acids on ADHD-related symptoms in children with specific learning difficulties. *Progress in Neuropsychopharmacology and Biological Psychiatry* **26**: 233-239.

Richardson, A.J., Cox, I.J., Sargentoni, J. and Puri, B.K. (1997). Abnormal cerebral phospholipid metabolism in dyslexia indicated by phosphorus-31 magnetic resonance spectroscopy. *NMR in Biomedicine* **10**: 309-314.

Richardson, A.J., Cyhlarova, E. and Puri, B.K. (2003). Clinical and biochemical fatty acid abnormalities in dyslexia, dyspraxia and schizotypy: an overview, in *Phospholipid Spectrum Disorder in Psychiatry and Neurology, 2nd edn.* (Peet, M., Glen, I. and Horrobin, D.F., eds.), Marius Press, Carnforth, Lancashire, pp. 477-490.

Ross, B.M., McKenzie, I., Glen, I. and Bennett, C.P. (2003). Increased levels of ethane, a non-invasive marker of n-3 fatty acid oxidation, in breath of children with attention deficit hyperactivity disorder. *Nutritional Neuroscience* **6**: 277-281.

Sacks, O. (1973). *Awakenings*. New York, USA: Vintage Books.

Stevens, L.J., Zhang, W., Peck, L., Kuczek, T., Grevstad, N., Mahon, A., Zentall, S.S., Arnold, L.E. and Burgess, J.R. (2003). EFA supplementation in children with inattention, hyperactivity, and other disruptive behaviors. *Lipids* **38**: 1007-1021.

Stevens, L.J., Zentall, S.S., Abate, M.L., Kuczek, T. and Burgess, J.R. (1996). Omega-3 fatty acids in boys with behavior, learning, and health problems. *Physiology and Behavior* **59**: 915-920.

Stevens, L.J., Zentall, S.S., Deck, J.L., Abate, M.L., Watkins, B.A., Lipp, S.R. and Burgess, J.R. (1995). Essential fatty acid metabolism in boys with attention-deficit hyperactivity disorder. *American Journal of Clinical Nutrition* **62**: 761-768.

Still, G.F. (1902). Some abnormal psychical conditions in children. *Lancet* **1**: 1008-1012, 1077-1082, 1163-1168.

Su, K.P., Huang, S.Y., Chiu, C.C. and Shen, W.W. (2003). Omega-3 fatty acids in major depressive disorder. A preliminary double-blind, placebo-controlled trial. *European Neuropsychopharmacology* **13**: 267-271.

Thorlaksdottir, A.Y., Skuladottir, G.V., Tryggvadottir, L., Stefansdottir, S., Hafsteinsdottir, H., Ogmundsdottir, H.O., Eyfjord, J.E., Jonsson, J.J. and Hardardottir, I. (2004). Positive association between DNA strand breaks in peripheral blood mononuclear cells and polyunsaturated fatty acids in red blood cells. *Abstracts of the*

Sixth Congress of the International Society for the Study of Fatty Acids and Lipids. Poster (4-5), page 129.

Thome, J. and Jacobs, K.A. (2004). Attention deficit hyperactivity disorder (ADHD) in a 19th century children's book. *European Psychiatry* **19**: 303-306.

Tredgold, A.F. (1908). *Mental Deficiency (Amentia)*. Baillière, Tindall and Cox: London, England.

Tredgold, A.F. (1952). *A Text-Book of Mental Deficiency (Amentia), 8th edition*. Baillière, Tindall and Cox: London, England.

Voigt, R.G., Llorente, A.M., Jensen, C.L., Fraley, J.K., Berretta, M.C. and Heird, W.C. (2001). A randomized, double-blind, placebo-controlled trial of docosahexaenoic acid supplementation in children with attention-deficit/hyperactivity disorder. *Journal of Pediatrics* **139**: 189-196.

World Health Organization (1992). *The ICD-10 Classification of Mental and Behavioural Disorders*. World Health Organization: Geneva.

Yamamoto, N., Saitoh, M., Moriuchi, A., Nomura, M. and Okuyama, H. (1987). Effect of dietary alpha linolenate/linoleate balance on brain lipid composition and learning ability in rats. *Journal of Lipid Research* **28**: 144-151.

Young, G.S., Maharaj, N.J. and Conquer, J.A. (2004). Blood phospholipid fatty acid analysis of adults with and without attention deficit/hyperactivity disorder. *Lipids* **39**: 117-123.

Zimmer, L., Vancassel, S., Cantagrel, S., Breton, P., Delamanche, S., Guilloteau, D., Durond, G. and Chalon, S. (2002). The dopamine mesocorticolimbic pathway is affected by deficiency in n-3 polyunsaturated fatty acids. *American Journal of Clinical Nutrition* **75**: 662-667.

Further sources of information

Recommended books

Barlow, W. (2001). *The Alexander Principle: How to Use Your Body without Stress*. London: Orion.

Gelb, M.J. (2004). *Body Learning: An Introduction to the Alexander Technique*. London: Aurum Press.

Graham, J. (1984). *Evening Primrose Oil: Its Remarkable Properties and its Use in the Treatment of a Wide Range of Conditions*. Wellingborough, Northamptonshire, U.K.: Thorsons Publishers Ltd.

Vogel, H.C.A. (1989). *The Nature Doctor*, 50th edition. Edinburgh: Mainstream Publishing.

Internet web sites

ADDISS.
This is the National Attention Deficit Disorder Information and Support Service. They provide information and resources about ADHD to parents, sufferers, teachers and health professionals.
www.addiss.co.uk

The British Dyslexia Association.
'The voice of dyslexic people. Our vision is that of a dyslexia friendly society that enables dyslexic people to reach their potential.'
www.bda-dyslexia.org.co.uk

Hyperactive Children's Support Group.
'Britain's leading proponent of a dietary approach to the problem of hyperactivity.'
www.hacsg.org.uk

Google.
Typing in attention deficit hyperactivity disorder or ADHD into the Google search engine will furnish you with some of the latest work in this area.
www.google.com

Dyspraxia Foundation.
'A UK charity that exists to help people to understand and cope with dyspraxia. A resourse for parents, teenagers and adults who have the condition and for professionals who help all of them.'
www.dyspraxiafoundation.org.uk

PubMed.
This allows you access to the abstracts of all recent medical and scientific research publications from international journals, without charge. Just type in the name of the authors (surname and then initial) and/or the subject area.
www.ncbi.nim.nih.gov/PubMed

VegEPA.
This is a good site for research and information about fatty acids and diseases such as ADHD. It also has information about mini-VegeCO, VegEPA and VegeCO. The product ordering line is 44 845 1300 424 from outside the UK, and 0845 1300 424 from within the UK.
www.vegepa.com

Useful names and addresses

ADDISS
10 Station Road
Mill Hill
London NW7 2JU
England, UK
Tel: 020 8906 9068
info@addiss.co.uk

ADHD.org.nz
c/o ADDvocate NZ Inc.
P.O. Box 249
Tauranga
NEW ZEALAND

BRITISH DYSLEXIA ASSOCIATION
98 London Road
Reading
RG1 5AU
Helpline: 0118 966 8271
helpline@bdadyslexia.org.uk

CHADD
8181 Professional Place
Suite 150
Landover

MD 20785
USA

DYSPRAXIA FOUNDATION
98 West Alley
Hitchin
Hertfordshire
SG5 1EG
Helpline: 01462 454 986
dyspraxia@dyspraxiafoundation.org.uk

THE HYPERACTIVE CHILDREN'S SUPPORT GROUP
71 Whyte Lane
Chichester
West Sussex
PO19 7DD
Tel: 01243 551 313
hyperactive@hacsg.org.uk

Mini-VegeCO and VegeCO manufacturer – see under VegEPA.

VegEPA manufacturer (also manufactures mini-VegeCO and VegeCO):
Igennus Ltd
St John's Innovation Centre
Cowley Road
Cambridge CB4 0WS
England, UK
Tel: +44 845 1300 424 from outside the UK, and 0845 1300 424 (low cost) from within the UK
www.vegepa.com

Index

A

AA, 81, 83, 88, 98, 99
academic achievement, 34–35
acne, 173
ADD – see attention deficit
    disorder
ADD/H – see attention deficit
    disorder
ADD/WO – see attention deficit
    disorder
Adderall – see dexamfetamine
adrenal gland, 158
adrenaline, 158
adrenoleucodystrophy, 36
air encephalography, 63
ALA, 81–82, 99
alcohol, 8, 41, 178
    effect on delta-6-
        desaturase, 87
Alexander Technique, 185
allergies, 8, 92–93
alpha-linolenic acid – see ALA
Aman, 107–108
American Academy of
    Neurology, 19
American Heart Association, 80
American Psychiatric Assoc-

iation, 29–30, 42–44
amfetamine – see amphetamine
amphetamine, 14, 19, 64, 65,
    70, 75
anaemia, 156, 157
antioxidant, 104
anxiety disorder, 35, 36
apoptosis, 91
apple oxidation, 103
arachidonic acid – see AA
arcus senilis, 168
Arnold, 108–109
aromatherapy, 188
arthralgia, 94
arthritis, 171–172
articulatory loop, 48
ascorbate, 159
ascorbic acid, 159
asthma, 7, 8, 93, 100
atomoxetine, 23, 24, 125,
    126–129
atrial fibrillation, 170–171
attention, 46–49
attention, deficit, 44, 45
attention deficit disorder, 43
Auster, Simon, 50
autistic spectrum disorder, 35
avidin, 159

Acknowledgements

Pages 18 to 21 The text and two illustrations are reproduced with permission from the DEA from the Congressional Testimony of Terrance Woodworth, the Deputy Director of the Office of Diversion Control of the United States Drug Enforcement Administration (DEA) before the Committee on Education and the Workforce: Subcommittee on Early Childhood Youth and Families on 16 May 2000.

Page 24 This extract is reproduced with permission from the Telegraph Group Ltd from the article by Celia Hall, Children's drug can cause liver damage, that appeared in the Daily Telegraph on 4 February 2005.

Pages 29 to 30 and page 40 The Diagnostic Criteria for AD/HD and for Developmental Coordination Disorder are reproduced with permission from the American Psychiatric Association from the Diagnostic and Statistical Manual of Mental Disorders, Fourth edition, Text Revision, Copyright 2000.

Page 31 The Diagnostic Criteria for Hyperkinetic Disorder are reproduced with permission from the World Health Organization from the ICD-10 Classification of Mental and Behavioural Disorders: Clinical Descriptions and Diagnostic Guidelines. Geneva, WHO 1992.

Page 32 This extract is taken from Quinn P and Wigal S (2004) Perceptions of girls and ADHD: results from a national survey. Medscape General Medicine volume 6(2), and is reproduced here with the permission of Medscape.

Pages 37 to 39 This material is reproduced with the permission of the publishers from Developmental Dyspraxia: identification and intervention: a manual for parents and professionals by Dr Madeleine Portwood, published by David Fulton, London, 1999.

Page 45 The Diagnostic Criteria for DAMP are reproduced from the article Hagberg B (1975) Minimal Brain Dysfunction. Lakartidningen volume 72, pages 3296 to 3300, with permission from the publisher and the author.

Page 48 Figure 3 is based on the working memory model described by Baddeley & Hitch in the book Bower GA (Editor) (1974) The Psychology of Learning and Motivation, volume 8. Academic Press, and is reproduced with the publisher's permission.

Page 51 The extracts from the Babylonian Talmud are reproduced from the 1938 translation published by Soncino Press, with permission from the publishers.

Pages 53 to 54 This extract is reproduced with permission from the publishers Elsevier, from the article Thome J & Jacobs KA (2004) Attention deficit hyperactivity disorder (ADHD) in a 19th century children's book, published in the European Journal of Psychiatry, volume 19, pages 303 to 306.

Page 65 This extract from the American Journal of Psychiatry 1937 (Bradley C., The behavior of children receiving Benzedrine, Volume 94, pages 577-585) is reprinted with the permission of the American Psychiatric Association.

Page 80 This extract is reprinted, ©2005, with the permission of the American Heart Association.

Pages 86, 90 to 91, and 109 These extracts are reprinted from Prostaglandins Leukotrienes & Essential Fatty Acids, volume 63, Richardson AJ & Puri BK, The potential role of fatty acids in attention-deficit/hyperactivity disorder, pages 79 to 87, Copyright 2000, with permission from Elsevier.

Pages 111 and 112 This extract is reprinted from Journal of Pediatrics, volume 139, Voigt RG et al, A randomised double-blind, placebo-controlled trial of docosahexaenoic acid supplementation in children with attention-deficit/hyperactivity disorder, pages 189 to 196, Copyright 2001, with permission from Elsevier.

Hammersmith Press titles from the same author

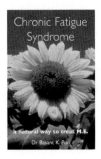

Chronic Fatigue Syndrome –
a natural way to treat M.E.
By Professor Basant K Puri
160pp £14.99
ISBN: 1-905140-00-2
Publication: January 2005

Whoever the ME sufferer, young or old, man or woman, he or she is likely to have been told the condition is 'psychosomatic' or 'all in the mind', depression is the root cause, and antidepressants the only sensible answer.

In this ground-breaking new book you will discover a very different way of looking at M.E. Professor Puri brings together historical and contemporary evidence to show how M.E. is almost certainly a physical, or 'organic' condition resulting from viral and other influences that reduce essential chemicals in the body. As such, it can be treated, and in a natural cost effective way

Read how and why EPA ('eicosapentaenoic acid') will be essential to recovery, how to take it, what supplements to have with it, and how to change to a lifestyle that will promote recovery.

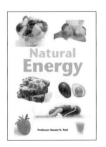

Natural Energy
By Professor Basant K Puri
224 pp £9.99
ISBN: 1-905140-02-9
Due for publication: January 2006

Extending the principles of treating M.E. and ADHD with a diet rich in phospholipids to the promotion of greater energy in any individual. Modern lifestyles are blamed for increasing tiredness experienced by the general population but poor diet has a significant role to play and there are clear ways to combat this trend and increase personal levels of physical and mental energy. Professor Puri explains what factors inhibit our bodies' healthy use of essential fatty acids and what factors do the reverse and why our ability to process omega-3 and omega-6 fatty acids effectively has such a profound effect on our health.

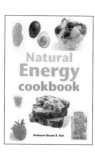

The Natural Energy Cookbook
By Professor Basant Puri
Cookery advisor: Sarah Banbery
224 pp £14.99
ISBN: 1-905140-03-7
Due for publication: February 2006

The practical way to achieve a diet high in phospho-lipids that is also delicious, varied and easy to prepare. Grouped around key ingredients, the book presents tried-and-tested recipes together with weekly menu plans. This is the 'how to do it' counterpart of 'Natural Energy', putting theory into practice in an attractively clear, and delicious, way.

Also from Hammersmith Press

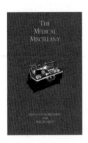

The Medical Miscellany
By Manoj Ramachandran & Max Ronson
174 pp £9.99
ISBN: 1-905140-05-3
Published 17 August 2005-07-26

This fascinating collection of medically-related items will inform, tantalize and infuriate you by turns. How can you tell if a murder victim was left- or right-handed? How many euphemisms can you think of for unmentionable parts of the body? What has chicken pox got to do with chickens? And does a famous doctor or medical scientist share your birthday?

We challenge you not to find something unexpected on every page, nor to smile or groan at almost every entry. How much do you know? How much will you be able to remember?

About the author

Professor Basant K. Puri
MA (Cantab), PhD, MB, BChir, BSc (Hons) MathSci, MRCPsych, DipStat, MMath

Professor Puri is Professor and Consultant at the MRI Unit, Imaging Sciences Department, MRC Clinical Sciences Centre, Hammersmith Hospital, London and Head of the Lipid Neuroscience Group, Imperial College London.

There have been two major studies to date which have been based on the ground-breaking use of omega-3 and omega-6 fatty acids to treat children with ADHD. The author has been involved in both of them. He also has a number of years' experience of successfully treating ADHD patients on an individual basis without the use of powerful stimulant medication.

Notes